AF825847

Second Edition

Medical Terminology

A LIVING LANGUAGE

Student Activity Guide

Bonnie F. Fremgen

Suzanne S. Frucht

Pearson

Cover art: Visuals Stock/Alamy Stock Photo; stockseller/123rf.com

Library of Congress Cataloging-in-Publication Data

Cataloging-in-Publication Data is available on file at the Library of Congress.

2 2023

Pearson

ISBN-10: 0-13-804578-X
ISBN-13: 978-0-13-804578-4

Contents

How to Use the Student Activity Guide xii

Chapter 1

Introduction to Medical Terminology

WORKSHEET 1A New Word Roots 2
WORKSHEET 1B New Prefixes 3
WORKSHEET 1C New Suffixes 5
WORKSHEET 1D Word Building Practice 7
WORKSHEET 1E Making Plurals 9
WORKSHEET 1F Medical Records 10
WORKSHEET 1G Unscramble. 11
WORKSHEET 1H Practice Building Medical Terms 12
WORKSHEET 1I Word Search Puzzle 13
WORKSHEET 1J Crossword Puzzle 14
QUIZ 1A New Word Parts Quiz. 16
QUIZ 1B Chapter Review. 17
QUIZ 1C Abbreviations Quiz. 19

Chapter 2

Body Organization

WORKSHEET 2A	New Combining Form	21
WORKSHEET 2B	Medical Term Analysis	24
WORKSHEET 2C	Unscramble	25
WORKSHEET 2D	Sound It Out	26
WORKSHEET 2E	Word Search Puzzle	27
WORKSHEET 2F	Crossword Puzzle	28
WORKSHEET 2G	Chapter Review	30
QUIZ 2A	New Word Parts Quiz	32
QUIZ 2B	Labeling Diagram	33
QUIZ 2C	Labeling Diagram	34
QUIZ 2D	Word Building Quiz	35
QUIZ 2E	Abbreviations Quiz	36
QUIZ 2F	Chapter Review	37

Chapter 3

Integumentary System

WORKSHEET 3A	New Combining Form, Prefix, and Suffix	40
WORKSHEET 3B	Medical Term Analysis	42
WORKSHEET 3C	Unscramble	43
WORKSHEET 3D	Sound It Out	44
WORKSHEET 3E	Word Search Puzzle	45

WORKSHEET 3F Crossword Puzzle 46
WORKSHEET 3G Chapter Review. 48
QUIZ 3A New Word Parts Quiz. 50
QUIZ 3B Labeling Diagram 51
QUIZ 3C Labeling Diagram 52
QUIZ 3D Word Building Quiz 53
QUIZ 3E Abbreviations Quiz. 54
QUIZ 3F Chapter Review. 55

Chapter 4

Musculoskeletal System

WORKSHEET 4A New Combining Form, Prefix, and Suffix 58
WORKSHEET 4B Medical Term Analysis 61
WORKSHEET 4C Unscramble. 62
WORKSHEET 4D Sound It Out 63
WORKSHEET 4E Word Search Puzzle 64
WORKSHEET 4F Crossword Puzzle 65
WORKSHEET 4G Chapter Review. 67
QUIZ 4A New Word Parts Quiz. 69
QUIZ 4B Labeling Diagram 70
QUIZ 4C Labeling Diagram 71
QUIZ 4D Word Building Quiz 72
QUIZ 4E Abbreviations Quiz. 73
QUIZ 4F Chapter Review. 74

Chapter 5

Cardiovascular System

WORKSHEET 5A New Combining Form and Suffix 77

WORKSHEET 5B Medical Term Analysis 79

WORKSHEET 5C Unscramble 80

WORKSHEET 5D Sound It Out 81

WORKSHEET 5E Word Search Puzzle 82

WORKSHEET 5F Crossword Puzzle 83

WORKSHEET 5G Chapter Review 85

QUIZ 5A New Word Parts 87

QUIZ 5B Labeling Diagram 88

QUIZ 5C Labeling Diagram 89

QUIZ 5D Word Building Quiz 90

QUIZ 5E Abbreviations Quiz 91

QUIZ 5F Chapter Review 92

Chapter 6

Blood and the Lymphatic and Immune Systems

WORKSHEET 6A New Combining Form and Suffix 95

WORKSHEET 6B Medical Term Analysis 97

WORKSHEET 6C Unscramble 98

WORKSHEET 6D Sound It Out 99

WORKSHEET 6E Word Search Puzzle 100

WORKSHEET 6F Crossword Puzzle . . . 101
WORKSHEET 6G Chapter Review. . . . 103
QUIZ 6A New Word Parts Quiz. . . . 105
QUIZ 6B Labeling Diagram . . . 106
QUIZ 6C Labeling Diagram . . . 107
QUIZ 6D Word Building Quiz . . . 108
QUIZ 6E Abbreviations Quiz. . . . 109
QUIZ 6F Chapter Review. . . . 110

Chapter 7

Respiratory System

WORKSHEET 7A New Combining Form and Suffix . . . 113
WORKSHEET 7B Medical Term Analysis . . . 115
WORKSHEET 7C Unscramble. . . . 116
WORKSHEET 7D Sound It Out . . . 117
WORKSHEET 7E Word Search Puzzle . . . 118
WORKSHEET 7F Crossword Puzzle . . . 119
WORKSHEET 7G Chapter Review. . . . 121
QUIZ 7A New Word Parts Quiz. . . . 124
QUIZ 7B Labeling Diagram . . . 125
QUIZ 7C Labeling Diagram . . . 126
QUIZ 7D Word Building Quiz . . . 127
QUIZ 7E Abbreviations Quiz. . . . 128
QUIZ 7F Chapter Review. . . . 129

Chapter 8

Digestive System

WORKSHEET 8A New Combining Form and Suffix 132
WORKSHEET 8B Medical Term Analysis 134
WORKSHEET 8C Unscramble. 135
WORKSHEET 8D Sound It Out 136
WORKSHEET 8E Word Search Puzzle 137
WORKSHEET 8F Crossword Puzzle 138
WORKSHEET 8G Chapter Review. 140
QUIZ 8A New Word Parts Quiz. 142
QUIZ 8B Labeling Diagram 143
QUIZ 8C Labeling Diagram 144
QUIZ 8D Word Building Quiz 145
QUIZ 8E Abbreviations Quiz. 146
QUIZ 8F Chapter Review. 147

Chapter 9

Urinary System

WORKSHEET 9A New Combining Form and Suffix 150
WORKSHEET 9B Medical Term Analysis 151
WORKSHEET 9C Unscramble. 152
WORKSHEET 9D Sound It Out 153
WORKSHEET 9E Word Search Puzzle 154

WORKSHEET 9F Crossword Puzzle 155
WORKSHEET 9G Chapter Review. 157
QUIZ 9A New Word Parts Quiz. 159
QUIZ 9B Labeling Diagram 160
QUIZ 9C Labeling Diagram 161
QUIZ 9D Word Building Quiz 162
QUIZ 9E Abbreviations Quiz. 163
QUIZ 9F Chapter Review. 164

Chapter 10

Reproductive System

WORKSHEET 10A New Combining Form, Suffix, and Prefix 167
WORKSHEET 10B Medical Term Analysis 170
WORKSHEET 10C Unscramble. 171
WORKSHEET 10D Sound It Out 172
WORKSHEET 10E Word Search Puzzle 173
WORKSHEET 10F Crossword Puzzle 174
WORKSHEET 10G Chapter Review. 176
QUIZ 10A New Word Parts Quiz. 178
QUIZ 10B Labeling Diagram 179
QUIZ 10C Labeling Diagram 180
QUIZ 10D Word Building Quiz 181
QUIZ 10E Abbreviations Quiz. 182
QUIZ 10F Chapter Review. 183

Chapter 11

Endocrine System

WORKSHEET 11A New Combining Form and Suffix 187
WORKSHEET 11B Medical Term Analysis 189
WORKSHEET 11C Unscramble. 190
WORKSHEET 11D Sound It Out 191
WORKSHEET 11E Word Search Puzzle 192
WORKSHEET 11F Crossword Puzzle 193
WORKSHEET 11G Chapter Review. 195
QUIZ 11A New Word Parts Quiz. 198
QUIZ 11B Labeling Diagram 199
QUIZ 11C Labeling Diagram 200
QUIZ 11D Word Building Quiz 201
QUIZ 11E Abbreviations Quiz. 202
QUIZ 11F Chapter Review. 203

Chapter 12

Nervous System and Mental Health

WORKSHEET 12A New Combining Form and Suffix 206
WORKSHEET 12B Medical Term Analysis 209
WORKSHEET 12C Unscramble. 210
WORKSHEET 12D Sound It Out 211
WORKSHEET 12E Word Search Puzzle 212

WORKSHEET 12F Crossword Puzzle 214
WORKSHEET 12G Chapter Review. 216
QUIZ 12A New Word Parts Quiz. 219
QUIZ 12B Labeling Diagram 220
QUIZ 12C Labeling Diagram 221
QUIZ 12D Word Building Quiz 222
QUIZ 12E Abbreviations Quiz. 223
QUIZ 12F Chapter Review. 224

Chapter 13

Special Senses: The Eye and Ear

WORKSHEET 13A New Combining Form and Suffix 227
WORKSHEET 13B Medical Term Analysis. 230
WORKSHEET 13C Scramble 231
WORKSHEET 13D Sound It Out 232
WORKSHEET 13E Word Search Puzzle 233
WORKSHEET 13F Crossword Puzzle 234
WORKSHEET 13G Chapter Review. 236
QUIZ 13A New Word Parts Quiz. 238
QUIZ 13B Labeling Diagram 239
QUIZ 13C Labeling Diagram 240
QUIZ 13D New Word Building Quiz. 241
QUIZ 13E Abbreviations Quiz. 242
QUIZ 13F Chapter Review. 243

How to Use the Student Activity Guide

The Student Activity Guide is designed to help you develop new skills and the knowledge necessary to work in nursing, medical assisting, radiology, or any other clinical aspect of medicine. It is an addition to the student text and guides you in learning to be a health care worker. Completing the activities and assignments reinforces your learning. Showing proficiency in skills gives you confidence when you begin your on-site training.

To use the Student Activity Guide most effectively:

- Carefully read each objective. Each objective tells you what you are expected to learn and to know.
- It is very difficult to "play catch-up." Complete the activities when they are assigned.
- Follow the directions. If you are instructed to complete an activity before reading, for example, be certain to complete it in the suggested order. Completing it helps you understand the reading material.
- Use your text to help you complete each activity assignment. The knowledge that you gain on the worksheet is important for passing the unit or chapter evaluation.
- Your instructor has the key for each activity. Check your answers for accuracy. If you have difficulty with answers, return to the text and read the information again. Do not move on until you are certain that you understand all concepts. Each concept builds on another. If you do not learn one concept, the next is more difficult to learn.

Chapter 1

Introduction to Medical Terminology

Learning Objectives

Upon completion of this chapter, you will be able to:

- Discuss the four parts of medical terms.
- Recognize word roots and combining forms.
- Identify the most common prefixes and suffixes.
- Define word building and describe a strategy for translating medical terms.
- State the importance of correct spelling of medical terms.
- State the rules for determining singular and plural endings.
- Discuss the importance of using caution with abbreviations.
- Recognize the documents found in a medical record.
- Recognize the different healthcare settings.
- Understand the importance of confidentiality.
- Describe how drugs are named and classified.
- Read and understand all abbreviations and notations in a written prescription.
- Understand reporting and recording medical information.
- Review healthcare teams.
- Recognize professional standards.

WORKSHEET 1A

New Word Roots

Directions: Write out the meaning for each of the following combining forms.

1. bi/o ______
2. carcin/o ______
3. cardi/o ______
4. chem/o ______
5. cis/o ______
6. dermat/o ______
7. enter/o ______
8. gastr/o ______
9. gynec/o ______
10. hemat/o ______
11. immun/o ______
12. laryng/o ______
13. nephr/o ______
14. neur/o ______
15. ophthalm/o ______
16. ot/o ______
17. path/o ______
18. pulmon/o ______
19. rhin/o ______

WORKSHEET 1B

New Prefixes

Directions: Write out the meaning of each of the following prefixes.

1. a- ______
2. an- ______
3. anti- ______
4. auto- ______
5. brady- ______
6. de- ______
7. dys- ______
8. endo- ______
9. epi- ______
10. eu- ______
11. ex- ______
12. extra- ______
13. hetero- ______
14. homo- ______
15. hyper- ______
16. hypo- ______
17. in- ______
18. inter- ______
19. intra- ______
20. macro- ______
21. micro- ______
22. neo- ______
23. para- ______
24. per- ______
25. peri- ______
26. post- ______

27. pre- ______________________________

28. pro- ______________________________

29. pseudo- ______________________________

30. re- ______________________________

31. retro- ______________________________

32. sub- ______________________________

33. tachy- ______________________________

34. trans- ______________________________

35. ultra- ______________________________

36. un- ______________________________

37. bi- ______________________________

38. hemi- ______________________________

39. mono- ______________________________

40. multi- ______________________________

41. nulli- ______________________________

42. pan- ______________________________

43. poly- ______________________________

44. quadri- ______________________________

45. semi- ______________________________

46. tetra- ______________________________

47. tri- ______________________________

WORKSHEET 1C

New Suffixes

Directions: Write out the meaning for each of the following suffixes.

1. -algia ______________________
2. -cele ______________________
3. -cyte ______________________
4. -dynia ______________________
5. -ectasis ______________________
6. -gen ______________________
7. -genic ______________________
8. -ia ______________________
9. -iasis ______________________
10. -ism ______________________
11. -itis ______________________
12. -logist ______________________
13. -logy ______________________
14. -lytic ______________________
15. -malacia ______________________
16. -megaly ______________________
17. -oma ______________________
18. -opsy ______________________
19. -osis ______________________
20. -pathy ______________________
21. -plasm ______________________
22. -plegia ______________________
23. -ptosis ______________________
24. -rrhage ______________________
25. -rrhagia ______________________
26. -rrhea ______________________

27. -rrhexis ____________________

28. -sclerosis ____________________

29. -stenosis ____________________

30. -therapy ____________________

31. -trophy ____________________

32. -centesis ____________________

33. -ectomy ____________________

34. -ostomy ____________________

35. -otomy ____________________

36. -pexy ____________________

37. -plasty ____________________

38. -rrhaphy ____________________

39. -tome ____________________

40. -gram ____________________

41. -graphy ____________________

42. -meter ____________________

43. -metry ____________________

44. -scope ____________________

45. -scopic ____________________

46. -scopy ____________________

WORKSHEET 1D

Word Building Practice

Directions: After each word part, write out its meaning. Then on the blank line, combine the word parts into a single word and write out its meaning.

1. gastr/o ________________

   -algia ________________

   ____

2. gynec/o ________________

   -logy ________________

   ____

3. nephr/o ________________

   -megaly ________________

   ____

4. pan- ________________

   cardi/o ________________

   -itis ________________

   ____

5. dys- ________________

   -plasia ________________

   ____

Directions: Break down each term into its word parts. Then write out the meaning of each word part. Finally, write out the meaning of the entire word.

6. rhinorrhea ____________________

____

7. carcinogenic ____________________

____

8. otoscope ____________________

____

9. hypertrophy ____________________

____

10. epigastric ____________________

____

WORKSHEET 1E

Making Plurals

Directions: Write the plural form for each singular term given below.

1. bursa ______________________________
2. thorax ______________________________
3. apex ______________________________
4. carcinoma ______________________________
5. diagnosis ______________________________
6. criterion ______________________________
7. bronchus ______________________________
8. diverticulum ______________________________
9. deformity ______________________________
10. larynx ______________________________

WORKSHEET 1F

Medical Records

Directions: Define each document found in a medical record in the space provided.

1. History and Physical ______________________________
2. Physician's Orders ______________________________
3. Nurse's Notes ______________________________
4. Physician's Progress Notes ______________________________
5. Consultation Reports ______________________________
6. Ancillary Reports ______________________________
7. Diagnostic Reports ______________________________
8. Informed Consent ______________________________
9. Operative Report ______________________________
10. Anesthesiologist's Report ______________________________
11. Pathologist's Report ______________________________
12. Discharge Summary ______________________________

WORKSHEET 1G

Unscramble

Directions: Unscramble each medical term below. A definition for the sought term is given below each scrambled term.

1. d o l o b ________________

   Meaning of combining form *hemat/o*

2. c o h a t s m ________________

   Meaning of combining form *gastr/o*

3. g i a t n a s ________________

   Meaning of prefix *anti-*

4. i t w u t o h ________________

   Meaning of prefix *an-*

5. w e t e b e n ________________

   Meaning of prefix *inter-*

6. l o m r n a ________________

   Meaning of prefix *eu-*

7. n i t a i l o d ________________

   Meaning of suffix *-ectasis*

8. a m l r e n t g e n ________________

   Meaning of suffix *-megaly*

9. g r a e d h n i n ________________

   Meaning of suffix *-sclerosis*

10. i a m o m f i a t n l n ________________

    Meaning of suffix *-itis*

WORKSHEET 1H

Practice Building Medical Terms

Directions: Use the word parts list below to build a medical term for each of the given definitions. In this exercise, some of the word parts are used more than once to illustrate how using the same word parts in different combinations produces terms with very different meanings.

Word Parts	Category	Meaning
-al	suffix	pertaining to
-ary	suffix	pertaining to
bronch/o	word root	bronchus
crani/o	word root	skull
-ectomy	suffix	surgical removal
intra-	prefix	within
-itis	suffix	inflammation
-logy	suffix	study of
neur/o	word root	nerve
-plasty	suffix	surgical repair
pulmon/o	word root	lung
-scope	suffix	instrument for viewing
tonsill/o	word root	tonsils

1. surgical removal of tonsils ______________/______________
2. study of the lungs ______________/______________/______________
3. pertaining to within the skull ______________/______________/______________
4. study of nerves ______________/______________/______________
5. surgical repair of the skull ______________/______________/______________
6. instrument for viewing the bronchus ______________/______________/______________
7. inflammation of the tonsils ______________/______________
8. inflammation of nerves ______________/______________
9. pertaining to within the lungs ______________/______________/______________
10. surgical repair of a bronchus ______________/______________/______________

WORKSHEET 1I

Word Search Puzzle

Directions: Find and circle the answer for each fill-in-the-blank question in the word search puzzle.

G	R	Q	L	F	X	F	B	G	N	T	V
E	B	H	K	Q	G	Q	N	T	N	F	B
S	P	B	C	K	F	I	V	C	P	E	K
A	D	N	N	G	W	R	L	W	T	S	Z
E	F	N	Y	O	L	L	E	W	J	L	D
S	X	E	R	D	H	N	E	C	K	O	X
I	K	R	N	C	R	E	R	V	O	W	J
D	A	Z	R	O	N	L	H	C	X	R	V
N	P	T	N	K	N	G	T	K	W	M	D
V	N	O	I	T	C	U	R	T	S	E	D
T	L	M	H	A	R	D	E	N	I	N	G
M	R	K	T	C	M	X	R	D	Y	K	M

1. The suffix *-pathy* means ______________________.
2. The suffix *-stenosis* means ______________________.
3. The suffix *-sclerosis* means ______________________.
4. The suffix *-gram* means ______________________.
5. The suffix *-lysis* means ______________________.
6. The prefix *brady-* means ______________________.
7. The prefix *inter-* means ______________________.
8. The prefix *nulli-* means ______________________.
9. The prefix *tri-* means ______________________.
10. The prefix *neo-* means ______________________.

WORKSHEET 1J

Crossword Puzzle

Directions: Use the definitions to complete the crossword puzzles. For all answers that are suffixes or prefixes, do not include the hyphen in your answer.

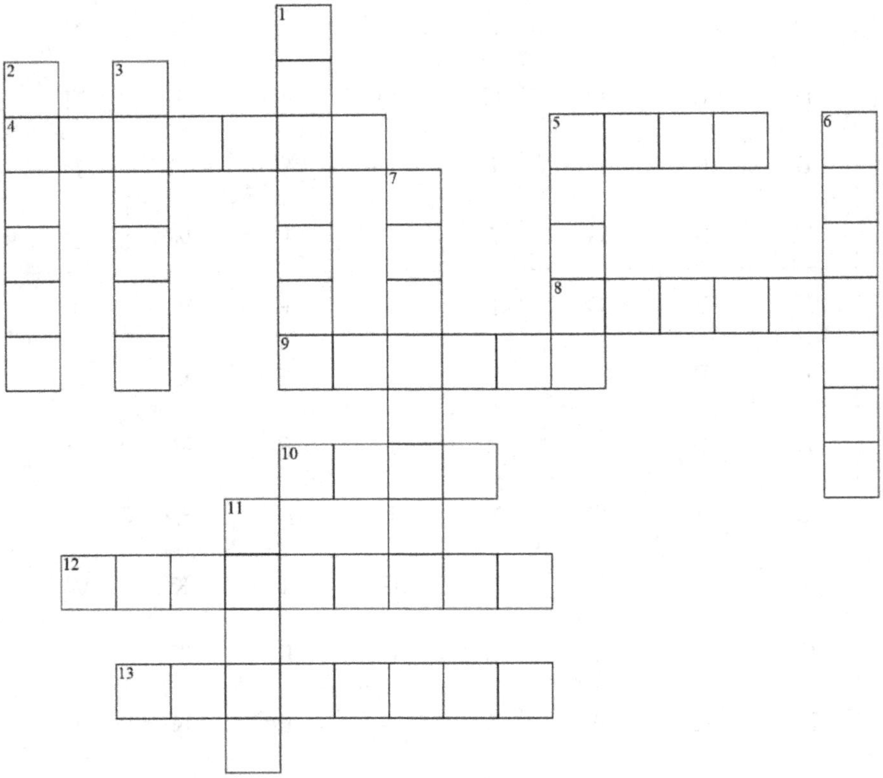

ACROSS

4 Treatment

5 brady-

8 Fear

9 Suffix meaning "surgical removal"

10 tachy-

12 Hardening

13 Narrowing

DOWN

1 -rrhexis

2 Drooping

3 Suffix meaning "enlargement"

5 Suffix meaning "visually examining"

6 Suffix meaning "abnormal softening"

7 Suffix meaning "puncture to withdraw fluid"

11 Suffix meaning "instrument for measuring"

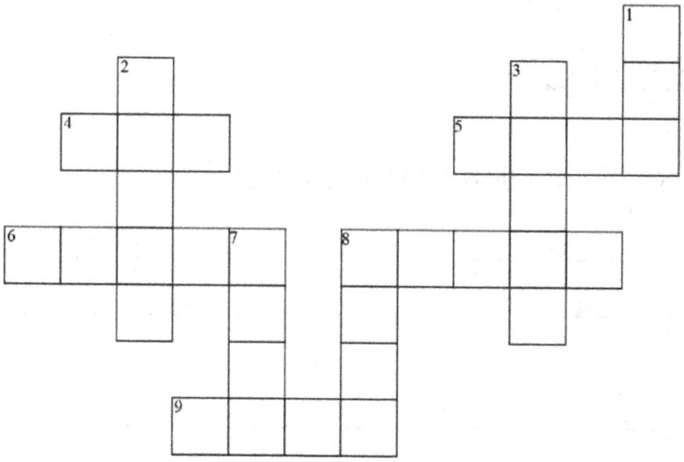

ACROSS

4. Beneath, under
5. Against
6. Inside, within
8. Excessive, above normal
9. One

DOWN

1. Above, upon
2. Many
3. Between
7. Self
8. Deficient, below normal

QUIZ 1A

New Word Parts Quiz

Directions: Define each of the following word parts.

1. cis/o ____________________
2. dermat/o ____________________
3. hemat/o ____________________
4. neur/o ____________________
5. pulmon/o ____________________
6. auto- ____________________
7. brady- ____________________
8. inter- ____________________
9. peri- ____________________
10. post- ____________________
11. trans- ____________________
12. eu- ____________________
13. poly- ____________________
14. hemi- ____________________
15. hypo- ____________________
16. -cyte ____________________
17. -osis ____________________
18. -malacia ____________________
19. -logy ____________________
20. -sclerosis ____________________
21. -rrhea ____________________
22. -ectomy ____________________
23. -ostomy ____________________
24. -scope ____________________
25. -metry ____________________

QUIZ 1B

Chapter Review

PART I: True/False

Directions: Write true or false to the right of each statement.

1. The word root is the foundation of a medical term. ____________________
2. The most common combining vowel is *i*. ____________________
3. Prefixes add meaning to a term such as a disease. ____________________
4. Many terms have alternate pronunciations. ____________________
5. Combining vowels are translated as "pertaining to." ____________________
6. Healthcare professionals have to be careful because some terms have the same beginning sound but are spelled differently. ____________________
7. Suffixes add meaning to a term such as a procedure. ____________________
8. A combining form is a word root and its suffix. ____________________
9. HIPAA sets federal standards to protect a patient's medical record. ____________________
10. Using one's own abbreviations is a good way to save time. ____________________
11. It is possible to build a medical term from only a prefix and a suffix. ____________________
12. The only word part found in every medical term is a word root. ____________________

PART II: Building Medical Terms

Directions: Fill in the blanks with the requested information.

1. In the term *otitis,* the suffix is , and this suffix means ____________________.
2. In the term *laryngectomy,* the word root is ____________________, and this word root means ____________________.
3. In the term *bradycardia,* the prefix is , and this prefix means ____________________.

4. Study the term *epigastric.*

What is the prefix and what does it mean? ______________________

____

What is the word root and what does it mean? ______________________

____

What is the suffix and what does it mean? ______________________

____

What does the entire term mean? ______________________

____

5. How many word roots are in the term *gastroenteritis*? ______________________

What are they? ______________________

____

6. Build a term for the phrase *abnormal softening of a nerve.* ______________________

____

7. Build a term for the phrase *discharge from the nose.* ______________________

____

8. Build a term for the phrase *study of the eye.* ______________________

____

9. Build a term for the phrase *gland tumor.* ______________________

____

10. Does the term built from *pulmon/o* and *-logy* require a combining vowel? ______________________

____

Explain your answer. ______________________

____

____

____

____

QUIZ 1C

Abbreviations Quiz

Directions: Write the medical term for which each abbreviation stands.

1. mg ______________________________

2. po ______________________________

3. Sig ______________________________

4. tid ______________________________

5. disp ______________________________

Chapter 2

Body Organization

Learning Objectives

Upon completion of this chapter, you will be able to:

- Recognize the combining forms introduced in this chapter.
- Correctly spell and pronounce medical terms and anatomical structures relating to body structure.
- Discuss the organization of the body in terms of cells, tissues, organs, and systems.
- Describe the common features of cells.
- Define the four types of tissues.
- List the major organs found in the 12 organ systems and their related medical specialties.
- Describe the anatomical position.
- Define the body planes.
- Identify regions of the body.
- List the body cavities and their contents.
- Locate and describe the nine anatomical and four clinical divisions of the abdomen.
- Define directional and positional terms.
- Build body organization medical terms from word parts.
- Interpret abbreviations associated with body organization.
- Describe routes used to introduce drugs into the body.

WORKSHEET 2A

New Combining Form

Directions: For each word part below, write its meaning. Then, locate a term from the chapter that uses the word part and its meaning.

Combining Forms	Meaning	Chapter Term	Meaning
1. abdomin/o			
2. adip/o			
3. anter/o			
4. bucc/o			
5. cardi/o			
6. caud/o			
7. cephal/o			
8. cervic/o			
9. chondr/o			
10. crani/o			
11. crin/o			
12. cutane/o			
13. cyt/o			
14. dermat/o			
15. dist/o			
16. dors/o			
17. enter/o			
18. epitheli/o			
19. gastr/o			
20. glute/o			
21. gynec/o			
22. hemat/o			
23. hist/o			

24. immun/o ______ ______ ______
25. infer/o ______ ______ ______
26. inguin/o ______ ______ ______
27. laryng/o ______ ______ ______
28. later/o ______ ______ ______
29. lumb/o ______ ______ ______
30. lymph/o ______ ______ ______
31. medi/o ______ ______ ______
32. muscul/o ______ ______ ______
33. nephr/o ______ ______ ______
34. neur/o ______ ______ ______
35. ophthalm/o ______ ______ ______
36. ot/o ______ ______ ______
37. orth/o ______ ______ ______
38. pariet/o ______ ______ ______
39. ped/o ______ ______ ______
40. pelv/o ______ ______ ______
41. peritone/o ______ ______ ______
42. pleur/o ______ ______ ______
43. poster/o ______ ______ ______
44. proct/o ______ ______ ______
45. proxim/o ______ ______ ______
46. pub/o ______ ______ ______
47. pulmon/o ______ ______ ______
48. rhin/o ______ ______ ______
49. spin/o ______ ______ ______
50. super/o ______ ______ ______
51. thorac/o ______ ______ ______
52. ur/o ______ ______ ______
53. urino/o ______ ______ ______

54. vascul/o ______________ ______________ ______________

55. ven/o ______________ ______________ ______________

56. vertebr/o ______________ ______________ ______________

57. viscer/o ______________ ______________ ______________

WORKSHEET 2B

Medical Term Analysis

Directions: Below are terms built from word parts used in this chapter. Many are built from word parts you have already learned. Analyze each term presented below. List and define the word parts used to build each term.

Medical Term	**Word Part Analysis**
1. cytology	______________________
2. cytoplasm	______________________
3. cardiac	______________________
4. adipose	______________________
5. abdominopelvic	______________________
6. pericardial	______________________
7. hypochondriac	______________________
8. epigastric	______________________
9. dermatology	______________________
10. intracavitary	______________________
11. otorhinolaryngology	______________________
12. gastroenterology	______________________
13. nephrology	______________________
14. parenteral	______________________
15. urology	______________________
16. neurology	______________________
17. ophthalmology	______________________
18. pulmonology	______________________
19. immunology	______________________
20. cardiology	______________________

WORKSHEET 2C

Unscramble

Directions: Unscramble each medical term below. A definition for the term is given below each scrambled term.

1. e m a l i d ______________________

   Refers to middle or near middle of body

2. p n u s i e ______________________

   Body lying horizontal and facing upward

3. a c r n i l a ______________________

   Cavity containing brain

4. e m r p t i n e o u ______________________

   Two-layered membrane in abdominopelvic cavity

5. s a t n s r v e e r ______________________

   Only horizontal body plane

6. p o e s r i y r a t r ______________________

   Body system containing the lungs

7. d a r r i u o c a a s c l v ______________________

   Body system containing the heart

8. y i r u a r n ______________________

   Body system containing the kidneys

9. t s i y o o h l g ______________________

   The study of tissues

10. n c o i e c t v e n ______________________

    Type of tissue that includes cartilage and bone

WORKSHEET 2D

Sound It Out

Directions: The following are some of the important terms from this chapter written as their phonetic spellings. Sound out each term and write it on the blank line.

1. sigh-TALL-oh-jee ______
2. ep-ih-THEE-lee-um ______
3. hiss-TALL-oh-jee ______
4. ADD-ih-pohs ______
5. in-teg-you-MEN-tah-ree ______
6. mus-qu-low-SKEL-et-all ______
7. car-dee-oh-VAS-kew-lar ______
8. gas-troh-en-ter-ALL-oh-jee ______
9. noo-RAL-oh-jee ______
10. SAJ-ih-tal ______
11. ab-DOM-ih-nal ______
12. SER-vih-kal ______
13. GLOO-tee-all ______
14. tho-RASS-ik ______
15. pair-ih-CAR-dee-al ______
16. VISS-er-ah ______
17. um-BILL-ih-kal ______
18. high-poh-GAS-trik ______
19. soo-PEE-ree-or ______
20. an-TEE-ree-or ______
21. in-FEE-ree-or ______
22. poss-TEE-ree-or ______
23. LAT-er-al ______
24. DISS-tal ______
25. MEE-dee-al ______

WORKSHEET 2E

Word Search Puzzle

Directions: Find and circle the answer for each fill-in-the-blank question in the word search puzzle.

G	J	L	M	Z	Z	T	H	R	F	V	L	Q
B	C	B	A	L	B	Q	C	G	L	A	M	Q
N	E	M	L	R	H	X	L	K	N	C	U	L
M	R	T	N	P	U	V	H	I	M	I	E	A
M	V	V	R	P	N	E	D	R	C	R	N	T
J	I	K	N	N	R	U	L	Q	Z	T	O	T
R	C	J	F	T	T	O	F	P	O	S	T	I
M	A	Y	Z	I	V	Z	N	R	M	A	I	G
Y	L	Q	G	T	B	M	B	E	D	G	R	A
R	T	N	L	W	T	I	R	J	M	I	E	S
K	O	F	J	N	T	G	K	M	Q	P	P	L
L	M	L	L	A	I	N	A	R	C	E	K	T
H	T	K	L	B	R	L	A	T	E	R	A	L

1. The ______________________ plane divides the body into left and right portions.
2. A ______________________ section is produced by a slice along the long axis of a structure.
3. ______________________ means "pertaining to the side."
4. ______________________ means "to lie face down."
5. ______________________ refers to the neck region of the body.
6. ______________________ refers to the eye socket region of the body.
7. The ______________________ cavity contains the brain.
8. Each of the ______________________ cavities contains a lung.
9. The anatomical division of the abdominopelvic cavity known as the ______________________ is the middle area of the upper row.
10. The ______________________ is a membrane covering that protects the abdominopelvic organs.

WORKSHEET 2F

Crossword Puzzle

Directions: Use the definitions to complete the crossword puzzles.

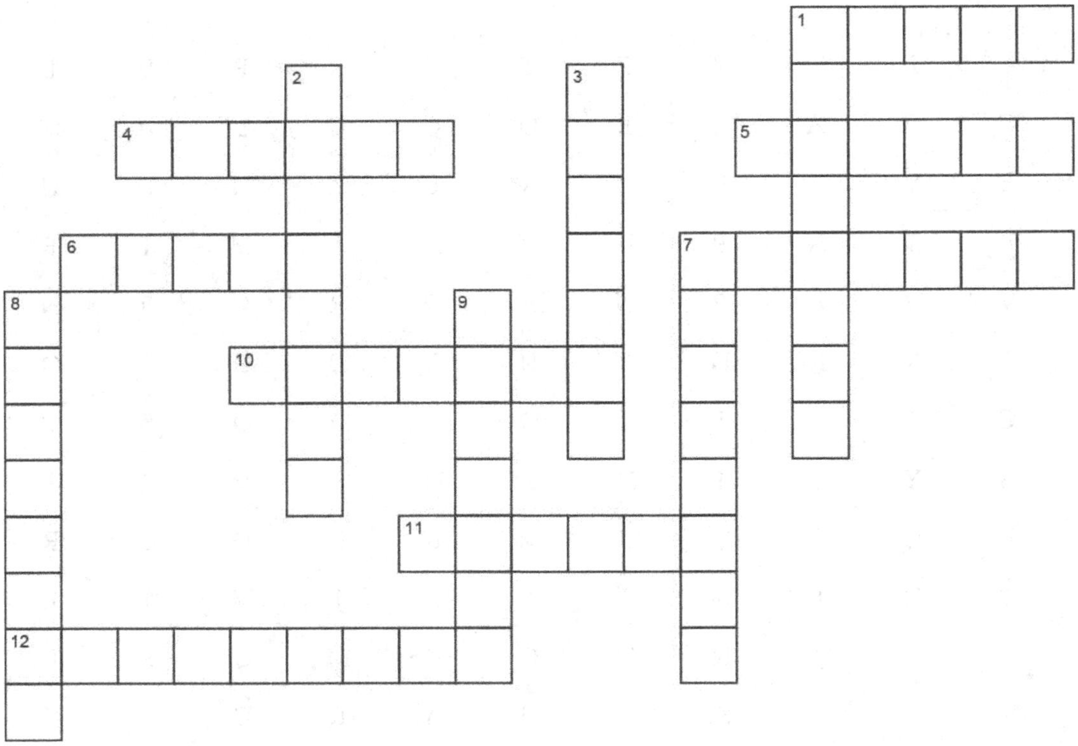

ACROSS

1 The neck connects the head to the ____________

4 Another name for the thoracic region

5 Term for posterior body region containing the back

6 Term for body region containing the genitals

7 Body cavity containing the brain

10 Referring to internal organs

11 Term for body region containing the leg

12 Term for anterior body region containing the abdomen

DOWN

1 Term for chest body region

2 Term for body region containing the arm

3 Term for posterior body region containing the buttocks

7 Term for body region containing the head

8 Term for neck body region

9 Direction term referring to the belly side of the body

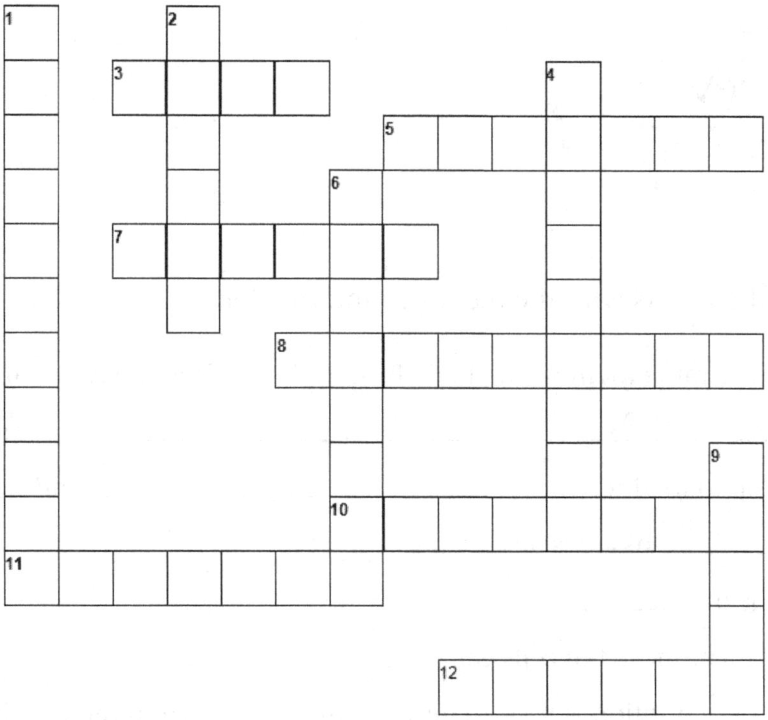

ACROSS

3 Direction term meaning "away from the surface"

5 Another name for frontal plane

7 Direction term referring to the tail

8 Separates thoracic and abdominal cavities

10 Direction term for front of body

11 Direction term referring to the side

12 Direction term meaning "to lie face up"

DOWN

1 Direction term meaning "nearer the surface"

2 Direction term referring to the middle

4 Direction term that means the same thing as dorsal

6 Plane that divides body into left and right portions

9 Direction term meaning "to lie face down"

WORKSHEET 2G

Chapter Review

Body Structure

Directions: Fill in the blanks with the requested information.

1. The hierarchical arrangement of the body from cells to whole body is cell, ____________________, ____________________, ____________________, and whole body.
2. All cells have the following: ________________, ________________, and ________________.
3. ____________________ tissue is designed to contract.
4. Adipose is a type of ____________________ tissue.
5. Nervous tissue is composed of cells called ____________________.
6. The______________ position is used to describe the positions and relationships of structures.
7. The ____________________ divides the thoracic cavity from the abdominopelvic cavity.
8. The pleural cavity contains the ____________________.
9. ____________________ tissue is composed of close-packed cells to form a covering.
10. ____________________ is the study of tissues.

Organs, Systems, and Medical Specialties

Directions: For each set of organs below, give the system they belong to and the medical specialty associated with that system.

Organs	System	Medical Specialty
1. skin, hair, nails	______________________________	______________________________
2. heart, blood vessels	______________________________	______________________________
3. lymph nodes, spleen	______________________________	______________________________
4. ungs, trachea	______________________________	______________________________
5. stomach, esophagus	______________________________	______________________________
6. kidneys, bladder	______________________________	______________________________
7. ovaries, uterus	______________________________	______________________________
8. testes, penis	______________________________	______________________________

9. thyroid, pituitary ______ ______

10. brain, nerves ______ ______

Matching

Directions: Match the term with its definition.

____ **1.** sagittal plane	**a.** Divides body into upper and lower portions
____ **2.** gluteal region	**b.** Top or summit of an organ
____ **3.** viscera	**c.** Buttocks
____ **4.** peritoneum	**d.** Central region of thoracic cavity
____ **5.** longitudinal section	**e.** Arm
____ **6.** thoracic region	**f.** A ventral cavity
____ **7.** spinal cavity	**g.** Neck
____ **8.** apex	**h.** Also the medial plane
____ **9.** transverse plane	**i.** Opposite direction from dorsal
____ **10.** pubic region	**j.** Membrane sac in abdominopelvic cavity
____ **11.** inferior	**k.** Lying face up
____ **12.** cervical region	**l.** Chest
____ **13.** brachial region	**m.** Slice along long axis of structure
____ **14.** anterior	**n.** Toward the belly side of the body
____ **15.** frontal plane	**o.** A dorsal cavity
____ **16.** supine	**p.** Torso
____ **17.** deep	**q.** Slice perpendicular to long axis of structure
____ **18.** thoracic cavity	**r.** Same direction as caudal
____ **19.** crural region	**s.** Head
____ **20.** mediastinum	**t.** Genital region
____ **21.** ventral	**u.** Further away from surface of body
____ **22.** cross-section	**v.** Divides body into front and back portions
____ **23.** trunk	**w.** Toward the side
____ **24.** lateral	**x.** Internal organs
____ **25.** cephalic region	**y.** Leg

QUIZ 2A

New Word Parts Quiz

Directions: Define the combining form in the spaces provided.

1. adip/o ______________________________
2. brachi/o ______________________________
3. caud/o ______________________________
4. cephal/o ______________________________
5. chondr/o ______________________________
6. crani/o ______________________________
7. cyt/o ______________________________
8. dist/o ______________________________
9. dors/o ______________________________
10. glute/o ______________________________
11. hist/o ______________________________
12. infer/o ______________________________
13. later/o ______________________________
14. medi/o ______________________________
15. neur/o ______________________________
16. oste/o ______________________________
17. pleur/o ______________________________
18. poster/o ______________________________
19. proxim/o ______________________________
20. pub/o ______________________________
21. vascul/o ______________________________
22. thorac/o ______________________________
23. ven/o ______________________________
24. viscer/o ______________________________
25. anter/o ______________________________

QUIZ 2B

Labeling Diagram

Directions: Label the planes of the body.

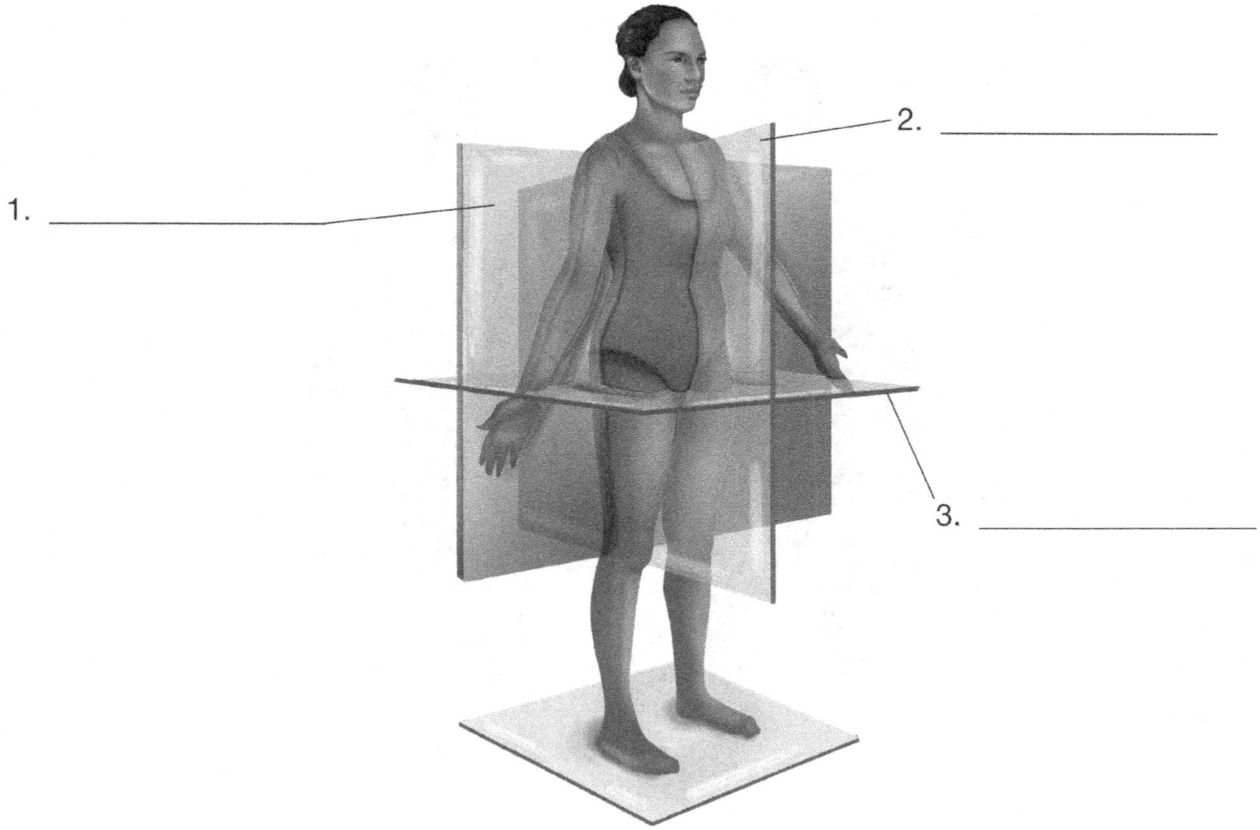

QUIZ 2C

Labeling Diagram

Directions: Label the regions of the body.

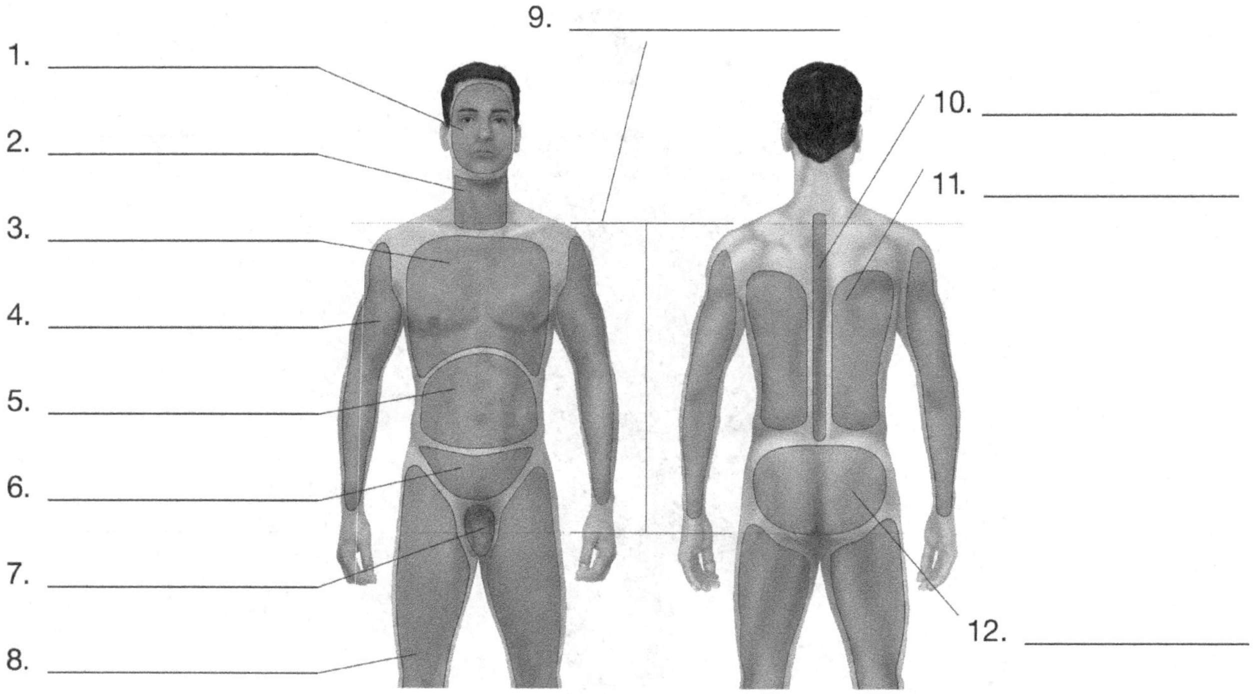

QUIZ 2D

Word Building Quiz

Directions: Build a single medical term for each phrase below.

1. pertaining to the abdomen ____________________
2. pertaining to the front ____________________
3. pertaining to the arm ____________________
4. pertaining to the head ____________________
5. pertaining to the neck ____________________
6. pertaining to the skull ____________________
7. pertaining to the leg ____________________
8. pertaining to the back of the body ____________________
9. pertaining to the epithelium ____________________
10. pertaining to the buttocks ____________________
11. pertaining to below ____________________
12. pertaining to the side ____________________
13. pertaining to the middle ____________________
14. pertaining to muscles ____________________
15. pertaining to heart and blood vessels ____________________
16. pertaining to blood ____________________
17. pertaining to the pelvis ____________________
18. pertaining to the genital region ____________________
19. pertaining to lymph ____________________
20. pertaining to the spine ____________________
21. pertaining to above ____________________
22. pertaining to the peritoneum ____________________
23. pertaining to the chest ____________________
24. pertaining to the belly side ____________________
25. pertaining to internal organs ____________________

QUIZ 2E

Abbreviations Quiz

Directions: Write the medical term for which each abbreviation stands.

1. AP ______________________________
2. CV ______________________________
3. ENT ______________________________
4. GI ______________________________
5. GYN ______________________________
6. lat ______________________________
7. LE ______________________________
8. LLQ ______________________________
9. LUQ ______________________________
10. MS ______________________________
11. OB ______________________________
12. PA ______________________________
13. RLQ ______________________________
14. RUQ ______________________________
15. UE ______________________________

QUIZ 2F

Chapter Review

PART I: Multiple Choice

Directions: Circle the correct answer.

1. Posterior is similar in meaning to
   - **a.** dorsal.
   - **b.** anterior.
   - **c.** ventral.
   - **d.** sagittal.
2. The body is divided into right and left sides by which of the following planes?
   - **a.** coronal
   - **b.** sagittal
   - **c.** transverse
   - **d.** frontal
3. The crural region is the
   - **a.** leg.
   - **b.** arm.
   - **c.** buttocks.
   - **d.** trunk.
4. The basic structural and functional unit of all living things is a(n)
   - **a.** organ.
   - **b.** nerve.
   - **c.** tissue.
   - **d.** cell.
5. Which is *not* an example of connective tissue?
   - **a.** stomach lining
   - **b.** bone
   - **c.** cartilage
   - **d.** adipose
6. Which is a visceral organ located in the thoracic cavity?
   - **a.** stomach
   - **b.** spleen
   - **c.** pancreas
   - **d.** heart
7. A structure located farthest from the surface of the body is
   - **a.** deep.
   - **b.** distal.
   - **c.** proximal.
   - **d.** superficial.
8. Which anatomical region of the abdominopelvic cavity is in the middle of the upper row?
   - **a.** hypochondriac
   - **b.** hypogastric
   - **c.** inguinal
   - **d.** epigastric

9. Which of the following does *not* describe an anatomical position?

a. lying face up
b. arms to the side
c. palms forward
d. toes pointing forward

10. Which route of administration involves a shallow injection just under the top layer of skin?

a. Parenteral
b. Intradermal
c. Intracavitary
d. Inhalation

PART II: Matching

Directions: Match the organ with its system.

_____ 1. stomach	a. female reproductive
_____ 2. skin	b. respiratory
_____ 3. uterus	c. endocrine
_____ 4. lungs	d. cardiovascular
_____ 5. bones	e. digestive
_____ 6. thyroid gland	f. male reproductive
_____ 7. brain	g. urinary
_____ 8. testes	h. musculoskeletal
_____ 9. heart	i. integumentary
_____ 10. bladder	j. nervous

PART III: Abbreviations

Directions: Write the full meaning of the following abbreviations.

1. lat ____________________
2. GYN ____________________
3. RUQ ____________________
4. LE ____________________

Chapter 3

Integumentary System

Learning Objectives

Upon completion of this chapter, you will be able to:

- Identify and define the combining forms, prefixes, and suffixes introduced in this chapter.
- Correctly spell and pronounce medical terms and major anatomical structures relating to the integumentary system.
- List and describe the four purposes of the skin.
- Describe the three layers of skin and the subcutaneous layer and their functions.
- List and describe the accessory organs of the skin.
- Identify and define integumentary system anatomical terms.
- Identify and define selected integumentary system pathology terms.
- Identify and define selected integumentary system diagnostic procedures.
- Identify and define selected integumentary system therapeutic procedures.
- Identify and define selected medications relating to the integumentary system.
- Define selected abbreviations associated with the integumentary system.

WORKSHEET 3A

New Combining Form, Prefix, and Suffix

Directions: For each word part below, write its meaning, and then locate a term from the chapter that uses the word part and its meaning.

Combining Forms	Meaning	Chapter Term	Meaning
1. albin/o			
2. cauter/o			
3. cry/o			
4. cutane/o			
5. derm/o			
6. dermat/o			
7. diaphor/o			
8. electr/o			
9. erythr/o			
10. hidr/o			
11. ichthy/o			
12. kerat/o			
13. leuk/o			
14. lip/o			
15. melan/o			
16. myc/o			
17. necr/o			
18. onych/o			
19. pedicul/o			
20. phot/o			
21. py/o			
22. rhytid/o			
23. sarc/o			
24. scler/o			

25. seb/o ______ ______ ______

26. system/o ______ ______ ______

27. trich/o ______ ______ ______

28. ungu/o ______ ______ ______

29. vesic/o ______ ______ ______

30. xer/o ______ ______ ______

Suffixes

31. -derma ______ ______ ______

Prefixes

32. allo- ______ ______ ______

33. xeno- ______ ______ ______

WORKSHEET 3B

Medical Term Analysis

Directions: Below are terms built from word parts used in this chapter. Some may use word parts you have not learned yet. In those cases, use the Appendices to translate those word parts. Analyze each term presented below, and list and define the word parts used to build each term.

Medical Term	Word Part Analysis
1. pediculosis	______________________
2. dermatology	______________________
3. hyperemia	______________________
4. keratosis	______________________
5. hemangioma	______________________
6. albinism	______________________
7. carcinoma	______________________
8. ichthyosis	______________________
9. onychia	______________________
10. biopsy	______________________
11. cytology	______________________
12. dermatome	______________________

WORKSHEET 3C

Unscramble

Directions: Unscramble each medical term below. A definition for the term is given below each scrambled term.

1. u p p l e a ______________________

   Solid, raised skin lesion

2. a l a c r i v e l ______________________

   Chickenpox

3. c y o s h e s m i c ______________________

   Black and blue skin bruise

4. r a g g e n n e ______________________

   Tissue necrosis

5. b t m i r e d n e e d ______________________

   Removal of dead or damaged tissue from wound

6. c o h c o l a m n a i a y ______________________

   Softening of the nails

7. e l i n o s ______________________

   General term for wound, injury, or abnormality

8. r e y h r h i d p o i s s ______________________

   Abnormal condition of excessive sweating

9. m a d e r g t o o l y ______________________

   Study of the skin

10. c u b e u s a t o u s n ______________________

    Pertaining to under the skin

WORKSHEET 3D

Sound It Out

Directions: The following are some of the important terms from this chapter written as their phonetic spellings. Sound out each term and write it in the blank.

1. on-ih-koh-my-KOH-sis ______
2. cry-oh-SER-jer-ee ______
   ah-BRAY-zhun ______
3. kon-TWO-shun ______
4. SIST ______
5. an-hi-DROH-sis ______
6. BYE-op-see ______
7. sell-you-LYE-tis ______
8. ULL-ser ______
9. ek-ih-MOH-sis ______
10. de-BREED-mint ______
11. AB-sess ______
12. ep-ih-DER-mal ______
13. FISH-er ______
14. high-poh-DER-mik ______
15. NOD-yool ______
16. MACK-yool ______
17. sklair-ah-DER-mah ______
18. neh-KROH-sis ______
19. der-mah-TALL-oh-jee ______
20. seb-or-EE-ah ______
21. sub-kyoo-TAY-nee-us ______
22. UNG-gwal ______
23. loo-koh-DER-mah ______

WORKSHEET 3E

Word Search Puzzle

Directions: Find and circle the answer for each fill-in-the-blank question in the word search puzzle.

L	L	Q	Q	L	A	G	N	U	F	T	S	M	D
L	A	P	T	K	W	V	K	R	B	I	Y	C	S
L	Q	L	X	T	X	T	V	Q	S	L	G	A	U
Q	B	K	O	N	B	P	N	E	G	B	O	U	T
L	M	K	N	P	R	V	R	M	A	J	L	T	I
K	T	N	B	T	E	O	A	M	Y	M	O	E	R
Z	Y	T	T	K	H	C	E	M	Y	J	T	R	U
N	G	R	Y	P	U	H	I	P	N	T	A	I	R
K	Y	R	A	L	T	F	T	A	R	M	M	Z	P
F	M	I	E	Y	C	O	M	E	D	O	R	A	L
L	D	T	R	Y	K	Q	L	J	R	M	E	T	X
R	W	E	K	V	P	B	L	F	N	Q	D	I	W
Y	G	D	E	R	M	A	B	R	A	S	I	O	N
T	L	W	C	H	J	L	P	W	K	R	N	N	X

1. ______________________ is the medical specialty that treats conditions of the skin.
2. The term ______________________ describes a red skin condition.
3. The medical term for a blackhead is ______________________.
4. ______________________ is a term that means profuse sweating.
5. ______________________ is the medical term meaning "baldness."
6. The intentional destruction of tissue by an electric current or a laser is called ____________.
7. ______________________ is a procedure used to remove acne scars.
8. A freckle and a birthmark are examples of a ______________________.
9. Tinea is a term to describe a ______________________ infection.
10. ______________________ means severe itching.

WORKSHEET 3F

Crossword Puzzle

Directions: Use the definitions to complete the crossword puzzles.

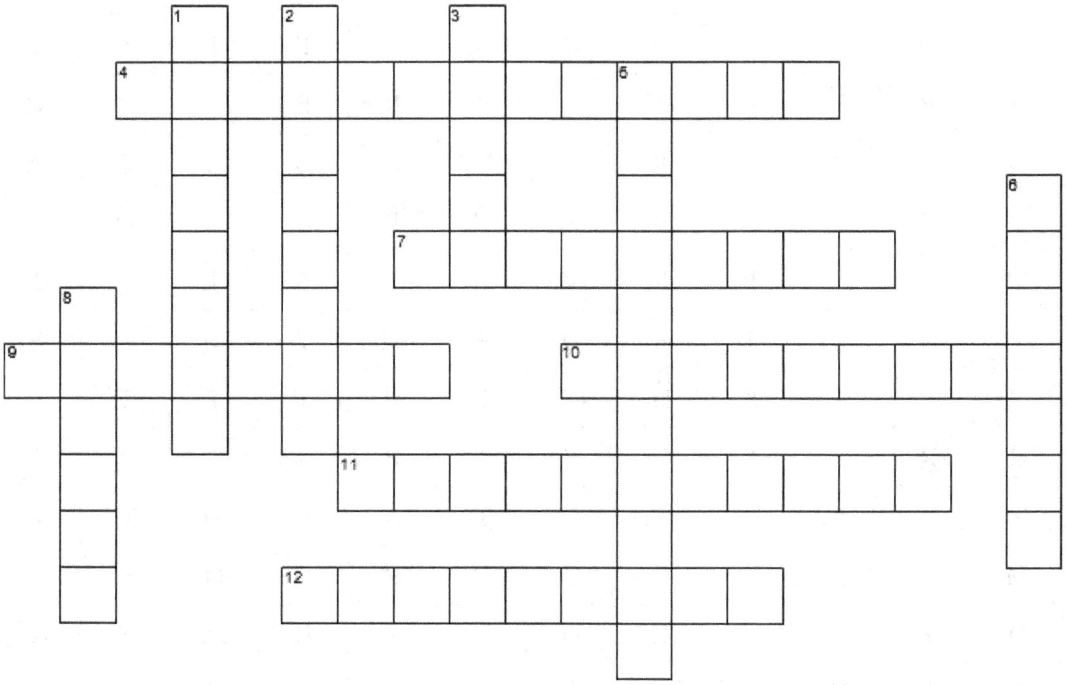

ACROSS

4 Term meaning "abnormal condition of excessive sweat"

7 Chickenpox

9 Disappearance of pigment from skin in patches

10 Term meaning "dry skin"

11 Term meaning "study of skin"

12 Outer layer of the skin

DOWN

1 Term describing blue skin

2 Area of tissue death

3 Fungal skin disease

5 Term meaning "surgical removal of nail"

6 Hard protein in hair and nails

8 Removal of a piece of tissue to examine with a microscope

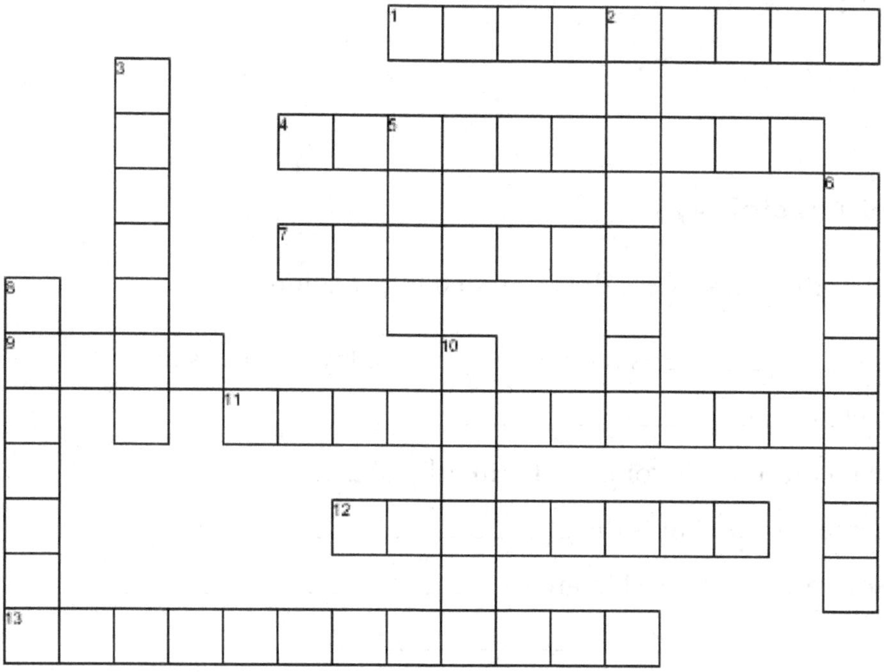

ACROSS

1 Instrument used to cut skin
4 "Black-and-blue" bruise
7 Crack-like break in the skin
9 Also called a furuncle
11 Also called a chemical peel
12 Severe itching
13 Term meaning "pertaining to under skin"

DOWN

2 Baldness
3 Inflamed nail bed
5 Fluid-filled sac under the skin
6 Term meaning "black tumor"
8 Localized collection of pus
10 Flat, discolored spot

WORKSHEET 3G

Chapter Review

Anatomy and Physiology

Directions: Fill in the blanks with the requested information.

1. The ____________________ is the most superficial layer of the skin.
2. Sebaceous glands secrete ____________________.
3. The subcutaneous layer is composed primarily of ____________________.
4. Another name for the skin is the ____________________ membrane.
5. The accessory organs of the skin are the____________________, ____________________, ____________________, and ____________________.
6. Sensory receptors are found in the ____________________ layer of the skin.
7. ____________________ is the pigment molecule that gives skin its color.
8. Hair and nails are composed of ____________________.
9. The ____________________ is the light-colored half-moon area at the base of the nail.
10. Sweat cools the skin by ____________________.

Word Building

Directions: Build a term for each of the following items.

1. surgical repair of the skin ____________________
2. black cell ____________________
3. softening of nails ____________________
4. oily discharge ____________________
5. scaly and dry skin ____________________
6. abnormal condition of hair fungus ____________________
7. abnormal condition of no sweat ____________________
8. pertaining to within the skin ____________________
9. skin inflammation ____________________
10. hard skin ____________________

Matching

Directions: Match the term with its definition.

_____ **1.** cicatrix	**a.** Hypertrophic scar
_____ **2.** diaphoresis	**b.** Remove tissue for diagnosis
_____ **3.** ecchymosis	**c.** Open sore
_____ **4.** keloid	**d.** Reduces severe itching
_____ **5.** purulent	**e.** Lice infestation
_____ **6.** ulcer	**f.** Mite infection
_____ **7.** vesicle	**g.** Leukoderma
_____ **8.** Kaposi's sarcoma	**h.** A scar
_____ **9.** decubitus ulcer	**i.** Baldness
_____ **10.** pediculosis	**j.** Removal of dead tissue from a wound
_____ **11.** varicella	**k.** Lab test to identify bacteria
_____ **12.** alopecia	**l.** Containing pus
_____ **13.** furuncle	**m.** Crack-like lesion on the skin
_____ **14.** vitiligo	**n.** Bacterial infection of hair follicle
_____ **15.** macule	**o.** Profuse sweating
_____ **16.** fissure	**p.** Powerful anti-inflammatory
_____ **17.** scabies	**q.** Chickenpox
_____ **18.** biopsy	**r.** Blister
_____ **19.** dermatoplasty	**s.** A bruise
_____ **20.** debridement	**t.** Cancer beginning in a melanocyte
_____ **21.** rhytidectomy	**u.** Flat, discolored spot on the skin
_____ **22.** corticosteroid cream	**v.** Skin cancer seen in AIDS patient
_____ **23.** antipruritic	**w.** Skin graft
_____ **24.** MM	**x.** Face lift
_____ **25.** C&S	**y.** Bedsore

QUIZ 3A

New Word Parts Quiz

Directions: Define the combining form or suffix in the spaces provided.

1. albin/o ____________________

2. cauter/o ____________________

3. kerat/o ____________________

4. lip/o ____________________

5. leuk/o ____________________

6. erythr/o ____________________

7. hidr/o ____________________

8. melan/o ____________________

9. necr/o ____________________

10. myc/o ____________________

11. seb/o ____________________

12. trich/o ____________________

13. xer/o ____________________

14. ungu/o ____________________

15. phot/o ____________________

16. py/o ____________________

17. scler/o ____________________

18. rhytid/o ____________________

19. albin/o ____________________

20. cutane/o ____________________

21. vesic/o ____________________

22. xer/o ____________________

23. -derma ____________________

24. allo- ____________________

25. xeno- ____________________

QUIZ 3B

Labeling Diagram

Directions: Label each of the skin structures on the figure below.

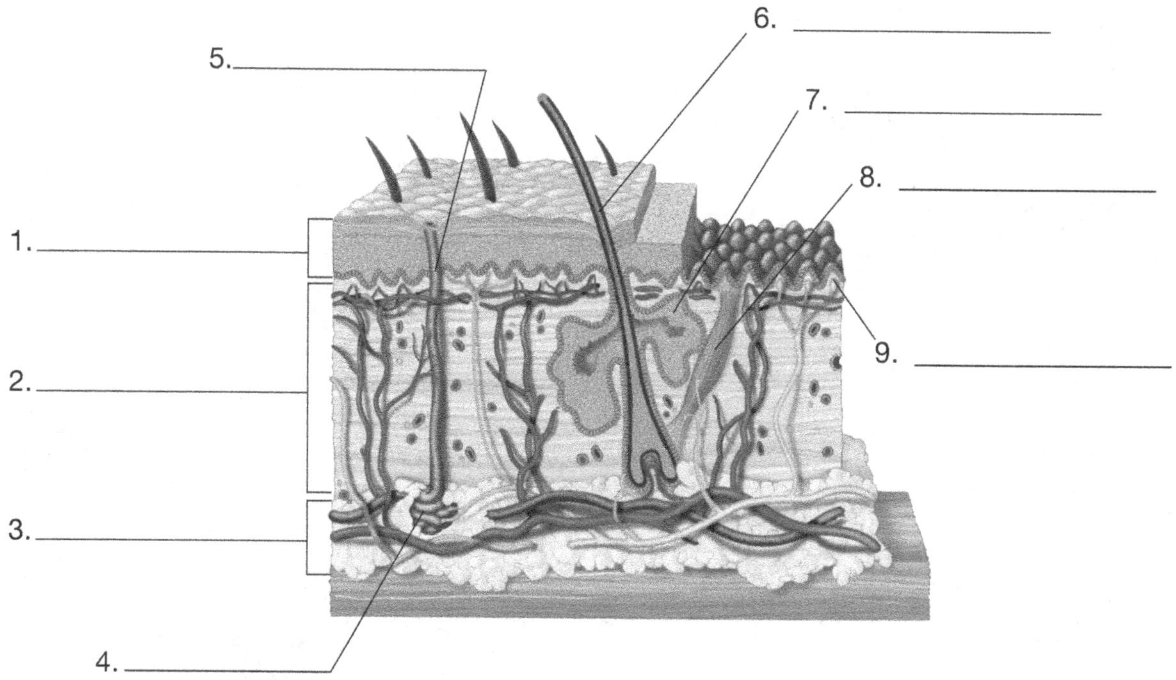

QUIZ 3C

Labeling Diagram

Directions: Label each of the internal structures of the skin on the figure below.

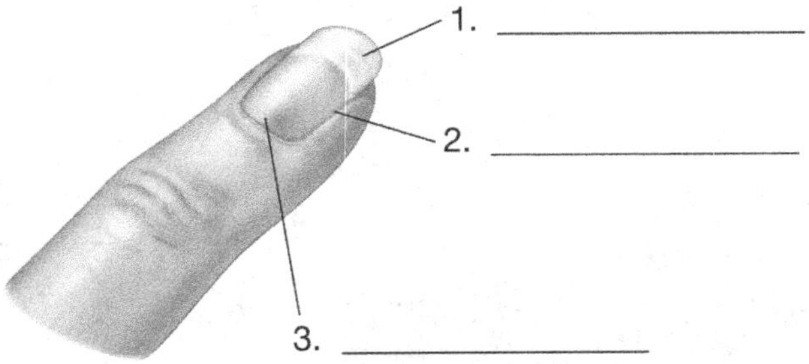

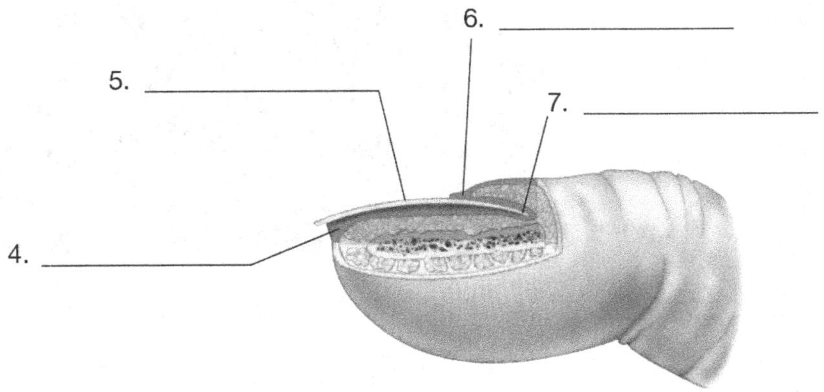

QUIZ 3D

Word Building Quiz

Directions: Build a single medical term for each of the phrases below.

1. surgical repair of skin ______
2. abnormal condition of no sweat ______
3. nail eating ______
4. abnormal condition of being blue ______
5. pertaining to nails ______
6. skin inflammation ______
7. study of skin ______
8. dry skin condition ______
9. hard skin condition ______
10. scaly and dry skin condition ______
11. red skin condition ______
12. oily discharge ______
13. abnormal condition of death ______
14. abnormal condition of excessive sweat ______
15. pertaining to within the skin ______
16. skin specialist ______
17. excessive blood condition ______
18. pertaining to under skin ______
19. fat mass ______
20. black cell ______
21. removal of nail ______
22. surgical removal of wrinkles ______
23. abnormal condition of hair fungus ______
24. pus skin condition ______
25. white skin condition ______

QUIZ 3E

Abbreviations Quiz

Directions: Write the medical term for which each abbreviation stands.

1. BCC ______
2. BX ______
3. C&S ______
4. decub ______
5. derm ______
6. FS ______
7. I&D ______
8. ID ______
9. MM ______
10. SCC ______
11. SG ______
12. SLE ______
13. STSG ______
14. subq ______
15. UV ______

QUIZ 3F

Chapter Review

PART I: Multiple Choice

Directions: Circle the correct answer.

1. A skin graft from one person to another is called a(n)
   - **a.** autograft.
   - **b.** homograft.
   - **c.** heterograft.
   - **d.** allograft.
2. The surgical procedure commonly called a face lift is a
   - **a.** rhytidectomy.
   - **b.** liposuction.
   - **c.** dermabrasion.
   - **d.** chemabrasion.
3. The viral skin infection commonly called German measles is
   - **a.** verruca.
   - **b.** varicella.
   - **c.** rubella.
   - **d.** scabies.
4. The sweat glands in the underarm and pubic area are called
   - **a.** sudoriferous glands.
   - **b.** sebaceous glands.
   - **c.** perspiration glands.
   - **d.** apocrine glands.
5. A skin discoloration or bruise caused by blood collecting under the skin is
   - **a.** ecchymosis.
   - **b.** erythema.
   - **c.** hirsutism.
   - **d.** acne.
6. Urticaria is the medical term for
   - **a.** ringworm.
   - **b.** lice.
   - **c.** hives.
   - **d.** ulcers.
7. The medical term for a dangerous form of skin cancer caused by an overgrowth of melanin-producing cells is
   - **a.** basal cell carcinoma.
   - **b.** Kaposi's sarcoma.
   - **c.** malignant melanoma.
   - **d.** squamous cell carcinoma.

8. A burn that damages the epidermis and dermis and causes redness and blisters is a

   a. first degree burn.
   b. second degree burn.
   c. third degree burn.
   d. fourth degree burn.

9. Build a medical term meaning *softening of the nail.*

   a. onychophagia
   b. rhytidectomy
   c. unguosis
   d. onychomalacia

10. Which medication is used to treat bacterial infections?

   a. antipruritic
   b. antibiotic
   c. antiseptic
   d. antiparasitics

PART II: Matching

Directions: Match the term with its definition.

_____ **1.** fissure	**a.** Fungal infection
_____ **2.** macule	**b.** Blister
_____ **3.** abscess	**c.** Crack-like lesion
_____ **4.** papule	**d.** Removal of lesion with a scraper
_____ **5.** vesicle	**e.** Mite infestation
_____ **6.** scabies	**f.** Flat, discolored spot
_____ **7.** tinea	**g.** Baldness
_____ **8.** varicella	**h.** Collection of pus
_____ **9.** alopecia	**i.** Small raised skin lesion
_____ **10.** curettage	**j.** Chickenpox

PART III: Abbreviations

Directions: Write the full meaning of the following abbreviations.

1. C&S ____________________
2. STSG ____________________
3. bx ____________________
4. I&D ____________________
5. derm ____________________

Chapter 4

Musculoskeletal System

Learning Objectives

Upon completion of this chapter, you will be able to:

- Identify and define the combining forms, prefixes, and suffixes introduced in this chapter.
- Correctly spell and pronounce medical terms and major anatomical structures relating to the musculoskeletal system.
- Locate and describe the major organs of the musculoskeletal system and their functions.
- Correctly place bones in either the axial or the appendicular skeleton.
- List and describe the components of a long bone.
- Identify bony projections and depressions.
- Identify the parts of a synovial joint.
- Describe the characteristics of the three types of muscle tissue.
- Use movement terminology correctly.
- Identify and define musculoskeletal system anatomical terms.
- Identify and define selected musculoskeletal system pathology terms.
- Identify and define selected musculoskeletal system diagnostic procedures.
- Identify and define selected musculoskeletal system therapeutic procedures.
- Identify and define selected medications relating to the musculoskeletal system.
- Define selected abbreviations associated with the musculoskeletal system.

WORKSHEET 4A

New Combining Form, Prefix, and Suffix

Directions: For each combining form, prefix, and suffix below, write its meaning. Then, locate a term from the chapter that uses the word part and its meaning.

Combining Forms	Meaning	Chapter Term	Meaning
1. ankyl/o			
2. arthr/o			
3. articul/o			
4. burs/o			
5. carp/o			
6. cervic/o			
7. chondr/o			
8. clavicul/o			
9. coccyg/o			
10. cortic/o			
11. cost/o			
12. crani/o			
13. femor/o			
14. fibul/o			
15. humer/o			
16. ili/o			
17. ischi/o			
18. kyph/o			
19. lamin/o			
20. lord/o			
21. lumb/o			
22. mandibul/o			
23. maxill/o			
24. medull/o			

25. metacarp/o ______ ______ ______
26. metatars/o ______ ______ ______
27. myel/o ______ ______ ______
28. orth/o ______ ______ ______
29. oste/o ______ ______ ______
30. patell/o ______ ______ ______
31. pector/o ______ ______ ______
32. ped/o ______ ______ ______
33. pelv/o ______ ______ ______
34. phalang/o ______ ______ ______
35. pod/o ______ ______ ______
36. prosthet/o ______ ______ ______
37. pub/o ______ ______ ______
38. radi/o ______ ______ ______
39. sacr/o ______ ______ ______
40. scapul/o ______ ______ ______
41. scoli/o ______ ______ ______
42. spin/o ______ ______ ______
43. spondyl/o ______ ______ ______
44. stern/o ______ ______ ______
45. synovi/o ______ ______ ______
46. synov/o ______ ______ ______
47. tars/o ______ ______ ______
48. thorac/o ______ ______ ______
49. tibi/o ______ ______ ______
50. uln/o ______ ______ ______
51. vertebr/o ______ ______ ______
52. duct/o ______ ______ ______
53. extens/o ______ ______ ______
54. fasci/o ______ ______ ______
55. fibr/o ______ ______ ______

56. flex/o ________ ________ ________
57. kinesi/o ________ ________ ________
58. muscul/o ________ ________ ________
59. my/o ________ ________ ________
60. myocardi/o ________ ________ ________
61. myos/o ________ ________ ________
62. plant/o ________ ________ ________
63. rotat/o ________ ________ ________
64. ten/o ________ ________ ________
65. tend/o ________ ________ ________
66. tendin/o ________ ________ ________
67. vers/o ________ ________ ________

Suffixes

68. –blast ________ ________ ________
69. -clasia ________ ________ ________
70. -desis ________ ________ ________
71. -listhesis ________ ________ ________
72. -logic ________ ________ ________
73. -porosis ________ ________ ________
74. -asthenia ________ ________ ________
75. -ion ________ ________ ________
76. -kinesia ________ ________ ________
77. -tonia ________ ________ ________
78. -trophic ________ ________ ________

Prefixes

79. ab- ________ ________ ________
80. ad- ________ ________ ________
81. circum- ________ ________ ________
82. e- ________ ________ ________

WORKSHEET 4B

Medical Term Analysis

Directions: Below are terms built from word parts used in this and previous chapters. Analyze each term presented below, and list and define the word parts used to build each term.

Medical Term **Word Part Analysis**

1. osteocyte ______
2. osteoblast ______
3. articular ______
4. kyphosis ______
5. scoliosis ______
6. orthotic ______
7. osteogenic ______
8. osteomalacia ______
9. osteoporosis ______
10. spondylolisthesis ______
11. osteoarthritis ______
12. systemic ______
13. arthrography ______
14. arthroscopy ______
15. arthroplasty ______
16. myoneural ______
17. electromyography ______
18. atrophy ______
19. pseudohypertrophic ______
20. fibromyalgia ______

WORKSHEET 4C

Unscramble

Directions: Unscramble each medical term below. A definition for the term is given below each scrambled term.

1. m r a o f e l ______

Pertaining to the thigh

2. l a t e a l p r ______

Pertaining to the knee cap

3. t a o s c l ______

Pertaining to a rib

4. b l a d i a n m u r ______

Pertaining to the lower jaw

5. p a c u s r a l ______

Pertaining to the shoulder blade

6. l u c v i l a r a c ______

Pertaining to the collar bone

7. l i s o c o i s s ______

Abnormal lateral curvature of the spine

8. p a r a i o r d h g y ______

maging procedure using x-rays

9. o c t u r a n r t e c ______

Abnormal shortening of muscle fibers

10. r t t o i o h c ______

Orthopedic appliance, such as a brace

WORKSHEET 4D

Sound It Out

Directions: The following are some of the important terms from this chapter written as their phonetic spellings. Sound out each term and write it in the blank.

1. figh-broh-my-AL-jee-ah ____________
2. brad-ee-kih-NEE-see-ah ____________
3. KON-droh-plas-tee ____________
4. mack-sih-LAIR-ree ____________
5. ee-lek-troh-MY-oh-gram ____________
6. sin-OH-vee-al ____________
7. FEM-or-all ____________
8. ILL-ee-ack ____________
9. in-ter-VER-teh-bral ____________
10. ber-SIGH-tis ____________
11. met-ah-CAR-pal ____________
12. FIB-yoo-lar ____________
13. ar-thro-sen-TEE-sis ____________
14. kray-nee-OTT-oh-mee ____________
15. my-oh-REK-sis ____________
16. oss-tee-oh-mi-ell-EYE-ti ____________
17. skoh-lee-OH-sis ____________
18. pa-TELL-ar ____________
19. pross-THEE-sis ____________
20. ray-dee-OG-rah-fee ____________
21. spon-dih-LOW-sis ____________
22. oss-tee-oh-por-ROH-sis ____________
23. ten-oh-DIN-ee-ah ____________
24. kon-TRACK-chur ____________

WORKSHEET 4E

Word Search Puzzle

Directions: Find and circle the answer for each fill-in-the-blank question in the word search puzzle.

W	C	O	M	P	R	E	S	S	I	O	N	G
S	A	I	S	A	L	C	O	R	H	T	R	A
T	I	R	G	M	A	L	R	C	T	N	N	Q
S	G	Q	R	S	I	R	E	K	Y	R	B	K
I	L	J	E	T	N	C	D	B	V	K	H	D
D	A	S	E	N	A	N	U	L	P	P	B	M
E	Y	I	N	E	R	Y	C	X	H	T	C	M
P	M	S	S	M	C	Q	T	L	R	K	U	M
O	O	O	T	A	A	F	I	D	K	N	L	M
H	R	H	I	G	R	N	O	K	R	P	V	C
T	B	P	C	I	T	H	N	E	B	J	Q	L
R	I	Y	K	L	N	G	T	F	C	G	B	F
O	F	K	M	Y	I	S	Y	N	D	J	M	P

1. The bones are joined together by ____________________ to form the skeleton.
2. Orthopedic surgeons are also referred to as ____________________.
3. The anatomical name for the breast bone is the ____________________.
4. ____________________ is a term meaning "to surgically break a joint."
5. ____________________ is a term meaning "inside the skull."
6. A ____________________ fracture results in loss of height of a vertebral body.
7. ____________________ is a chronic condition with widespread aching and pain in the muscles and fibrous soft tissue.
8. A ____________________ fracture is commonly seen in children.
9. An abnormal increase in the normal outward curvature of the thoracic spine is called ____________________.
10. ____________________ means to realign the bones in a fracture or dislocation.

WORKSHEET 4F

Crossword Puzzle

Directions: Use the definitions to complete the crossword puzzles.

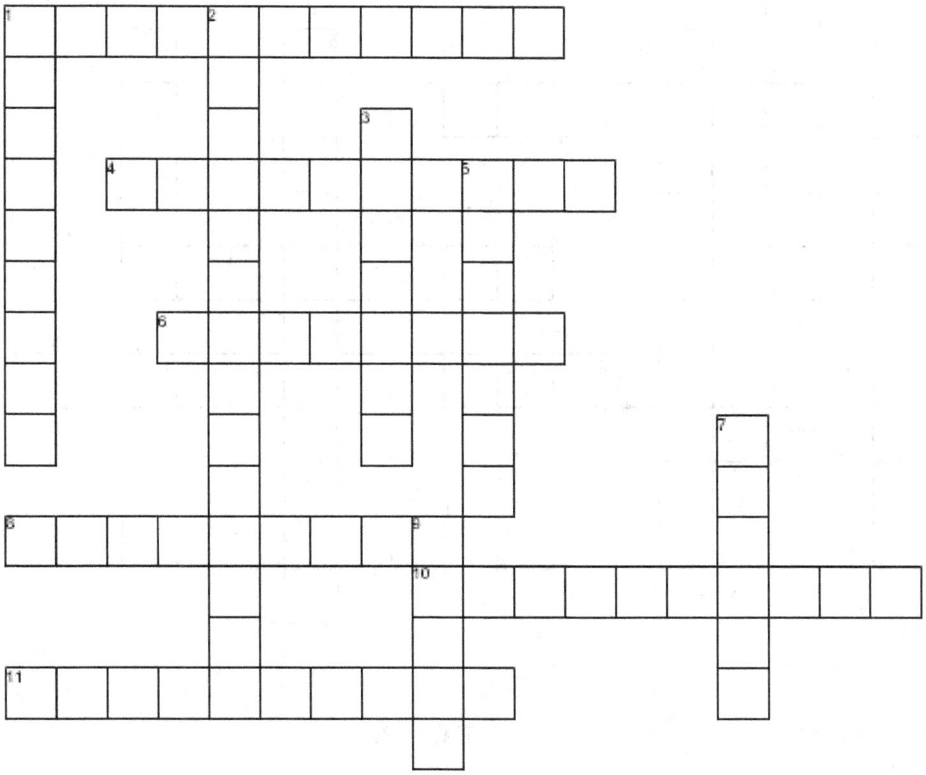

ACROSS

1 Imaging procedure using X-rays

4 ____________________ arthritis is an autoimmune disease

6 Externally applied brace or splint

8 Abnormal lateral curvature of the spine

10 Artificial device used to substitute for a missing body part

11 Fracture with a line straight across the shaft of bone

DOWN

1 Procedure to correct fracture by realigning bone

2 Arthritis caused by loss of cartilage cushion covering bone

3 Osteogenic ____________________ is the most common type of bone cancer

5 An ____________________ fracture line runs on an angle to the bone shaft

7 Slight fracture caused by repetitive low-impact forces

9 Sudden, involuntary, strong muscle contraction

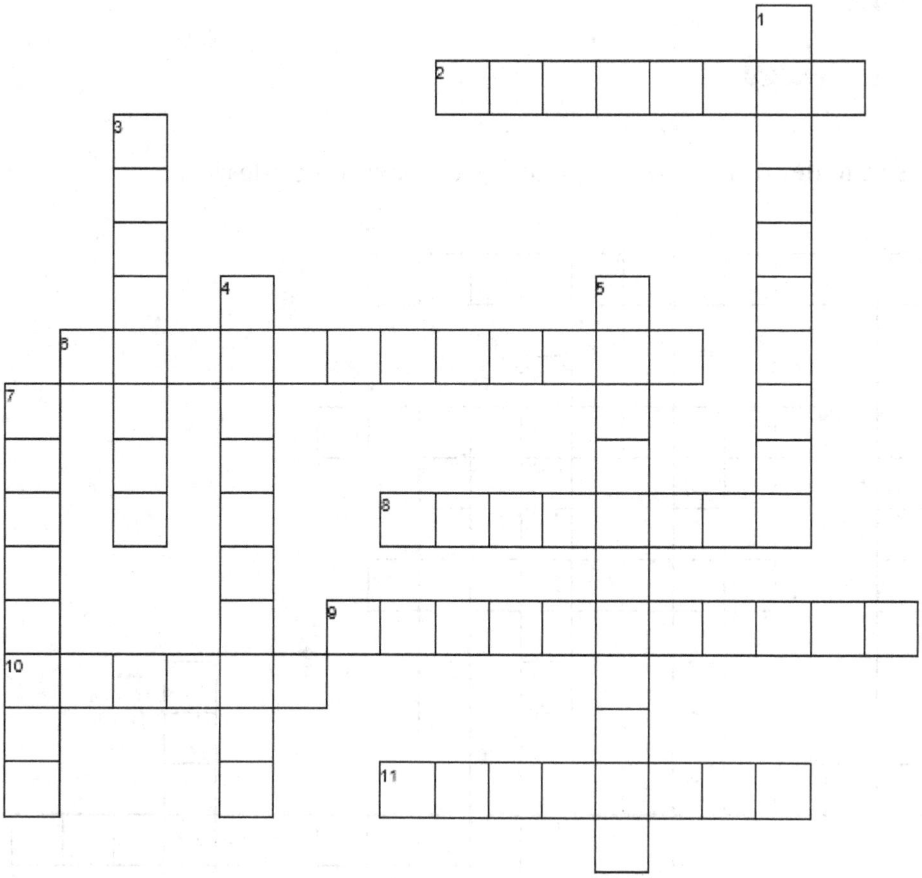

ACROSS

2 Procedure to stabilize fractured bone

6 Chronic condition with widespread muscle aching and pain

8 Fracture in which broken bone causes open skin wound

9 Abnormal shortening of muscle fibers

10 Damage to the muscles or tendons from overstretching

11 Medical term for swayback

DOWN

1 Fracture with shattered bone

3 Anatomical name for the lower jaw

4 Fracture with incomplete break

5 Joint is displaced from normal alignment

7 Medical term for hunchback

WORKSHEET 4G

Chapter Review

Anatomy and Physiology

Directions: Fill in the blanks with the requested information.

1. The four classifications of bones by their shape are ____________________, ____________________, ____________________, and ____________________.
2. Dense and hard exterior surface bone is called ______________ or ______________ bone.
3. A(n) ________________ is a large, smooth, ball-shaped process on the end of a long bone.
4. The bones that form the central axis for the whole body are part of the ________________ skeleton.
5. The pectoral girdle consists of the ____________________ and ____________________.
6. The most common type of joint in the body is a ____________________ joint.
7. Visceral muscle is another name for ____________________ muscle.
8. ____________________ muscles are voluntary.
9. ____________________ is movement away from the midline.
10. A(n) ____________________ anchors a muscle to a bone.

Word Building

Directions: Build a term for each of the following items.

1. cartilage softening ____
2. fusion of a joint ____
3. pertaining to between vertebrae ____
4. bone and cartilage tumor ____
5. pertaining to the femur ____
6. pertaining to the breast bone ____
7. lack of tone ____
8. study of movement ____
9. incision into fascia ____
10. record of muscle electricity ____

Matching

Directions: Match the term with its definition.

_____ **1.** clavicle	**a.** Brace or splint
_____ **2.** phalanges	**b.** Realigning bones in a fracture
_____ **3.** exostosis	**c.** Fracture commonly seen in children
_____ **4.** orthotic	**d.** Procedure to stabilize a joint
_____ **5.** comminuted	**e.** Loss of bone mass
_____ **6.** greenstick	**f.** Abnormal shortening of muscle fibers
_____ **7.** HNP	**g.** Bone spur
_____ **8.** subluxation	**h.** Sudden, strong muscle contraction
_____ **9.** RA	**i.** Fracture with shattered bone
_____ **10.** spina bifida	**j.** Wryneck
_____ **11.** osteoporosis	**k.** Noise from two bones rubbing together
_____ **12.** prosthesis	**l.** Inherited muscle degeneration disease
_____ **13.** crepitation	**m.** Considered an autoimmune disease
_____ **14.** DXA	**n.** Damage to ligaments around a joint
_____ **15.** reduction	**o.** Fingers
_____ **16.** NSAIDs	**p.** Aching and pain in muscles and soft tissue
_____ **17.** contracture	**q.** Collarbone
_____ **18.** spasm	**r.** Scar tissue in the fascia
_____ **19.** fibromyalgia	**s.** Device to substitute a missing body part
_____ **20.** carpal tunnel syndrome	**t.** Protruding intervertebral disk
_____ **21.** torticollis	**u.** Provide mild pain relief
_____ **22.** adhesion	**v.** Measures bone density
_____ **23.** MD	**w.** Congenital anomaly
_____ **24.** sprain	**x.** A repetitive motion disorder
_____ **25.** tenodesis	**y.** Incomplete dislocation

QUIZ 4A

New Word Parts Quiz

Directions: Define the combining form or suffix in the spaces provided.

1. arth/o ______________________________

2. carp/o ______________________________

3. cost/o ______________________________

4. lord/o ______________________________

5. scoli/o ______________________________

6. medull/o ______________________________

7. myel/o ______________________________

8. lumb/o ______________________________

9. thorac/o ______________________________

10. spondyl/o ______________________________

11. fasci/o ______________________________

12. myos/o ______________________________

13. plant/o ______________________________

14. tend/o ______________________________

15. kinesi/o ______________________________

16. fibr/o ______________________________

17. my/o ______________________________

18. synovi/o ______________________________

19. orth/o ______________________________

20. circum- ______________________________

21. -tonia ______________________________

22. -asthenia ______________________________

23. -desis ______________________________

24. -clasia ______________________________

25. -listhesis ______________________________

QUIZ 4B

Labeling Diagram

Directions: Label the bones of the skeleton.

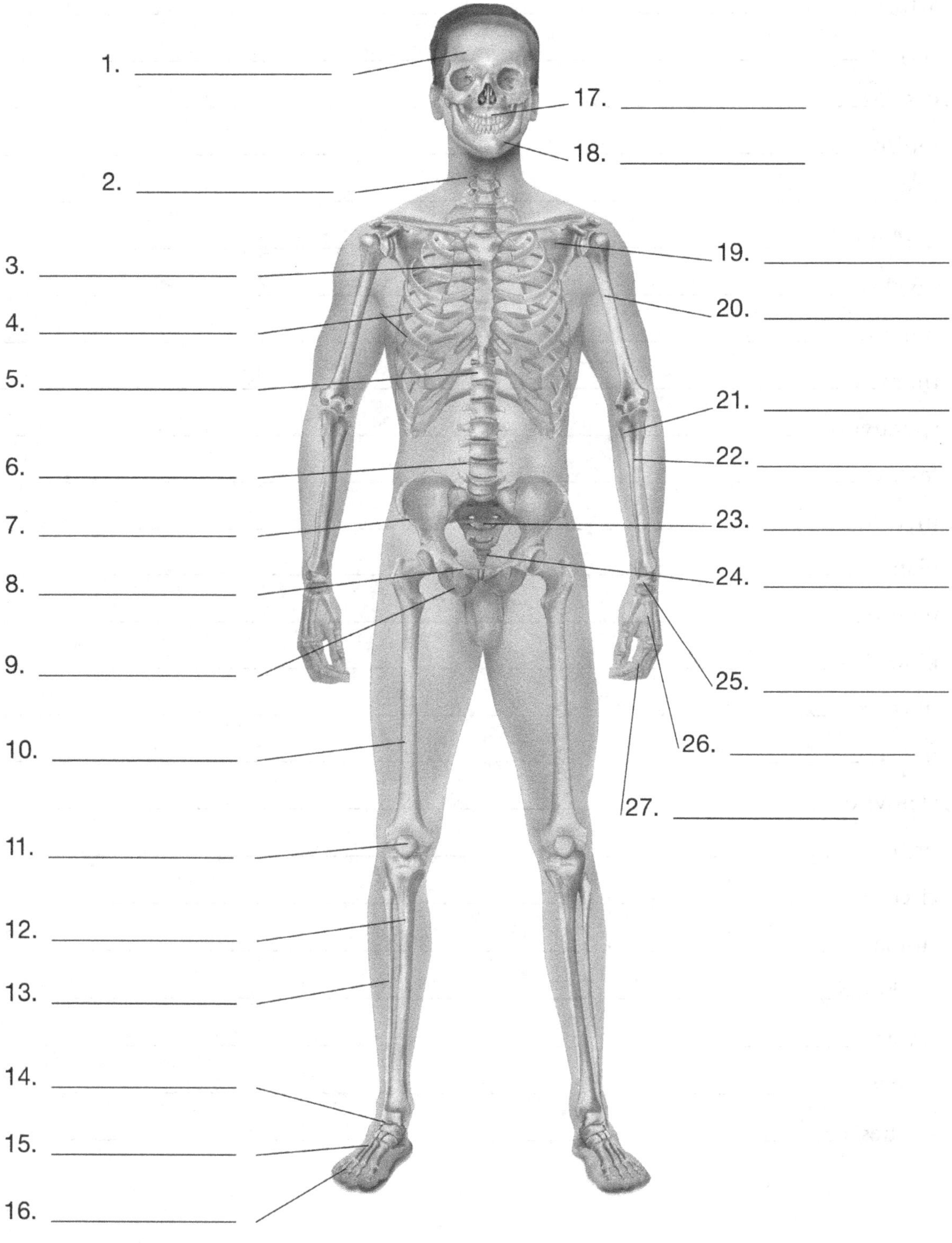

QUIZ 4C

Labeling Diagram

Directions: Label the parts of a long bone.

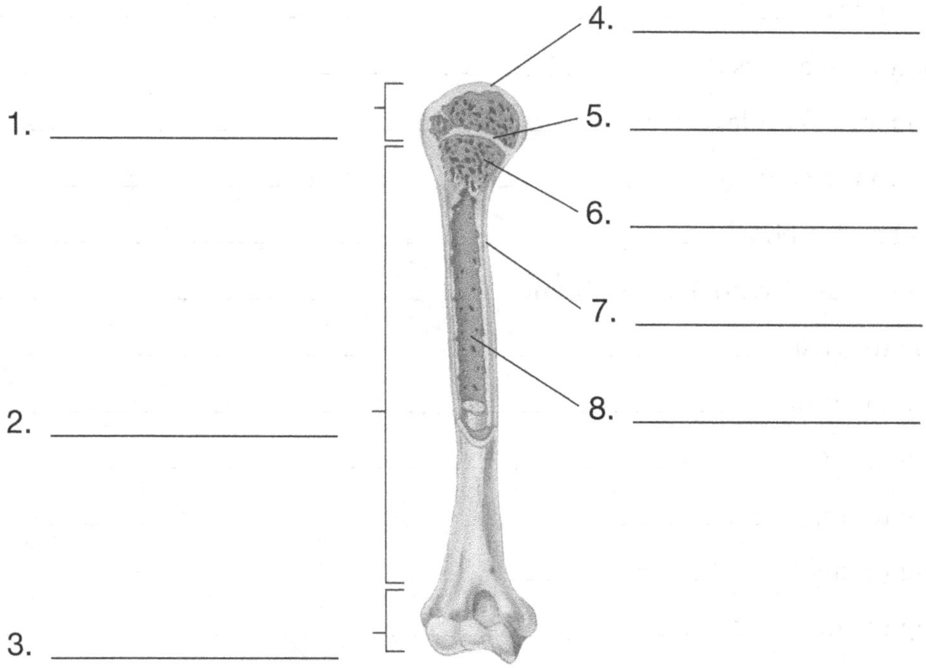

QUIZ 4D

Word Building Quiz

Directions: Build a single medical term for each phrase below.

1. fusion of a joint ______
2. inflammation of a bursa ______
3. surgical repair of cartilage ______
4. incision into the skull ______
5. surgically break a bone ______
6. surgical removal of synovial membrane ______
7. pertaining to wrist ______
8. pertaining to ilium ______
9. pertaining to kneecap ______
10. pertaining to upper jaw ______
11. pertaining to tailbone ______
12. pertaining to chest ______
13. abnormal condition of hump ______
14. porous bone ______
15. vertebra slipping ______
16. inflammation of bone and joint ______
17. process of recording a joint ______
18. inflammation of fascia ______
19. pertaining to muscle ______
20. muscle disease ______
21. inflammation of many muscles ______
22. abnormal tone ______
23. slow movement ______
24. excessive development ______
25. inflammation of a tendon ______

QUIZ 4E

Abbreviations Quiz

Directions: Write the medical term for which each abbreviation stands.

1. AE ______________________________
2. BK ______________________________
3. BDT ______________________________
4. DJD ______________________________
5. DXA ______________________________
6. Fx ______________________________
7. HNP ______________________________
8. NSAID ______________________________
9. ORIF ______________________________
10. RA ______________________________
11. THA ______________________________
12. TKR ______________________________
13. UE ______________________________
14. LE ______________________________
15. ortho ______________________________
16. JRA ______________________________
17. Ca ______________________________
18. L1 ______________________________
19. C2 ______________________________
20. T2 ______________________________
21. MD ______________________________
22. IM ______________________________
23. EMG ______________________________
24. DTR ______________________________
25. CTS ______________________________

QUIZ 4F

Chapter Review

PART I: Multiple Choice

Directions: Circle the correct answer.

1. The medical term for the end region of a long bone is

a. diaphysis.
b. epiphysis.
c. periosteum.
d. bursa.

2. Which bone is *not* found in the appendicular skeleton?

a. tibia
b. phalanges
c. clavicle
d. sternum

3. Most of the joints found in the human body are what type?

a. bursa joints
b. ball-and-socket joints
c. synovial joints
d. suture joints

4. The medical term for a fracture that does not break through the skin is

a. closed.
b. complete.
c. comminuted.
d. compound.

5. The term meaning "movement toward the midline" is

a. abduction.
b. circumduction.
c. eversion.
d. adduction.

6. A specialist in treating disorders of the feet is a(n)

a. orthopedist.
b. orthotist.
c. podiatrist.
d. physiatrist.

7. An inherited disease causing progressive muscle weakness and atrophy is

a. myasthenia.
b. carpal tunnel syndrome.
c. rheumatoid arthritis.
d. muscular dystrophy.

8. The medical term for the removal of muscle tissue for pathological examination is

a. myelography.
b. muscle biopsy.
c. dual-energy absorptiometry.
d. polymyositis.

9. The surgical term *arthrodesis* is defined as

   a. surgical fusion of a joint.
   b. surgical breaking of a joint.
   c. incision into a joint.
   d. excision of a joint.

10. The condition that involves an abnormal lateral curve of the spine is

   a. lordosis.
   b. ankylosis.
   c. kyphosis.
   d. scoliosis.

PART II: Matching

Directions: Match the term with its definition.

____ 1. fixation	a. procedure that uses radioactive dye
____ 2. laminectomy	b. fracture at an angle to the bone
____ 3. bone scan	c. muscle wasting
____ 4. osteoarthritis	d. stabilizing a broken bone while it heals
____ 5. talipes	e. tennis elbow
____ 6. oblique	f. clubfoot
____ 7. Colles'	g. forms on a tendon sheath
____ 8. atrophy	h. results in degeneration of bones and joints
____ 9. lateral epicondylitis	i. wrist fracture
____ 10. ganglion	j. used to correct severe back problems

PART III: Abbreviations

Directions: Write the full meaning of the following abbreviations.

1. DXA ____________________
2. C2 ____________________
3. RUE ____________________
4. DTR ____________________
5. OA ____________________

Chapter 5

Cardiovascular System

Learning Objectives

Upon completion of this chapter, you will be able to:

- Identify and define the combining forms, suffixes, and prefixes introduced in this chapter.
- Correctly spell and pronounce medical terms and major anatomical structures relating to the cardiovascular system.
- Describe the major organs of the cardiovascular system and their functions.
- Describe the anatomy of the heart.
- Describe the flow of blood through the heart.
- Explain how the electrical conduction system controls the heartbeat.
- List and describe the characteristics of the three types of blood vessels.
- Define pulse and blood pressure.
- Identify and define cardiovascular system anatomical terms.
- Identify and define selected cardiovascular system pathology terms.
- Identify and define selected cardiovascular system diagnostic procedures.
- Identify and define selected cardiovascular system therapeutic procedures.
- Identify and define selected medications relating to the cardiovascular system.
- Define selected abbreviations associated with the cardiovascular system.

WORKSHEET 5A

New Combining Form and Suffix

Directions: For each word part below, write its meaning. Then, locate a term from the chapter that uses the word part and its meaning.

Combining Forms	Meaning	Chapter Term	Meaning
1. angi/o	________	________	________
2. aort/o	________	________	________
3. arteri/o	________	________	________
4. ather/o	________	________	________
5. atri/o	________	________	________
6. cardi/o	________	________	________
7. coron/o	________	________	________
8. corpor/o	________	________	________
9. embol/o	________	________	________
10. isch/o	________	________	________
11. myocardi/o	________	________	________
12. phleb/o	________	________	________
13. sept/o	________	________	________
14. son/o	________	________	________
15. sphygm/o	________	________	________
16. steth/o	________	________	________
17. thromb/o	________	________	________
18. valv/o	________	________	________
19. valvul/o	________	________	________
20. varic/o	________	________	________
21. vascul/o	________	________	________
22. vas/o	________	________	________
23. ven/o	________	________	________
24. ventricul/o	________	________	________

Suffixes

25. –cardia ______ ______ ______

26. –manometer ______ ______ ______

27. –ole ______ ______ ______

28. –spasm ______ ______ ______

29. –tension ______ ______ ______

30. –tonic ______ ______ ______

31. –ule ______ ______ ______

Prefixes

32. di- ______ ______ ______

WORKSHEET 5B

Medical Term Analysis

Directions: Below are terms built from word parts used in this and previous chapters. Analyze each term presented below, and list and define the word parts used to build it.

Medical Term	Word Part Analysis
1. pulmonary	______
2. atrioventricular	______
3. cardiology	______
4. arteriosclerosis	______
5. atherosclerosis	______
6. hypotension	______
7. thrombophlebitis	______
8. angiography	______
9. valvulitis	______
10. electrocardiography	______
11. cardiopulmonary	______
12. thrombolytic	______
13. sphygmomanometer	______
14. cardiomyopathy	______
15. myocarditis	______
16. hypertension	______
17. intracoronary	______

WORKSHEET 5C

Unscramble

Directions: Unscramble each medical term below. A definition for the term is given below each scrambled term.

1. a i h m r t y ______________________

   Irregular heartbeat

2. i t p n o p a i l t a ______________________

   Racing heartbeat

3. a e i m h s c ______________________

   Loss of blood supply from occlusion

4. o l b n i l i a t i f r ______________________

   Abnormal quivering of the heart

5. y r e s o n e i n t p h ______________________

   High blood pressure

6. r a c y a b d i d ______________________

   Abnormally slow heart rate

7. m n u e r s a y ______________________

   A weakened and widened artery

8. r o c a y n ______________________

   Pertaining to the heart

9. l r e a r i t r o c e o s i s ______________________

   Hardening of an artery

10. m k a c e a e r p ______________________

    Electrical device to stimulate the heart to beat

WORKSHEET 5D

Sound It Out

Directions: The following are some of the important terms from this chapter written as their phonetic spellings. Sound out each term and write it in the blank.

1. AN-jee-oh-plas-tee ______________________
2. in-trah-VEE-nus ______________________
3. ath-er-oh-skleh-ROH-sis ______________________
4. brad-ee-CAR-dee-ah ______________________
5. CAR-dee-ak ______________________
6. CAR-dee-oh-VAS-kyoo-lar ______________________
7. ay-OR-tik ______________________
8. KOR-ah-nair-ee ______________________
9. ee-lek-troh-car-dee-OG-rah-fee ______________________
10. ul-trah-son-OG-rah-fee ______________________
11. is-KEYH-mee-ah ______________________
12. em-boh-LIZ-em ______________________
13. end-ar-teh-REK-toh-mee ______________________
14. fih-brill-AY-shun ______________________
15. high-per-TEN-shun ______________________
16. IN – farkt ______________________
17. VEE-nus ______________________
18. my-oh-CAR-dee-all ______________________
19. fleh-BYE-tis ______________________
20. in-ter-ven-TRIK-yoo-lar ______________________
21. VAL-view-lar ______________________
22. car-dee-oh-MEG-ah-lee ______________________
23. pol-ee-ar-ter-EYE-tis ______________________
24. throm-BOH-sis ______________________
25. STETH-oh-scope ______________________

WORKSHEET 5E

Word Search Puzzle

Directions: Find and circle the answer for each definition in the word search puzzle.

R	L	H	D	R	K	M	R	G	C	K	T	N	E	R	V
Q	H	M	N	G	D	K	R	Z	M	H	S	T	N	E	F
B	Z	L	N	M	L	N	Z	J	Y	M	I	J	D	T	Q
M	R	K	G	M	K	F	M	P	R	L	G	C	A	E	N
L	B	A	X	T	Y	Z	O	K	M	M	O	I	R	M	O
F	N	Z	D	J	N	T	L	M	N	M	L	T	T	O	I
C	M	T	D	Y	E	G	S	R	R	C	O	Y	E	N	T
N	G	F	F	N	C	Y	X	N	N	N	I	L	R	A	A
B	L	B	S	F	R	A	F	F	G	P	D	O	E	M	L
T	N	I	Q	U	C	V	R	W	T	M	R	B	C	O	L
L	O	V	E	H	B	B	Q	D	R	T	A	M	T	M	I
N	L	N	K	G	M	G	H	L	I	C	C	O	O	G	R
Q	A	L	L	L	Q	K	K	N	R	A	C	R	M	Y	B
T	B	M	J	H	C	J	Z	M	P	V	K	H	Y	H	I
L	Y	R	T	T	C	R	A	F	N	I	L	T	R	P	F
T	V	A	R	R	H	Y	T	H	M	I	A	N	L	S	L

1. A specialist in studying the heart ______________________
2. A localized widening of an artery ______________________
3. An irregular heartbeat ______________________
4. An abnormally slow heartbeat ______________________
5. Surgical removal of the inner lining of an artery ______________________
6. Abnormal quivering of the heart ______________________
7. A decrease in blood pressure ______________________
8. An area of tissue necrosis ______________________
9. Drug that dissolves existing blood clot ______________________
10. A blood pressure cuff ______________________

WORKSHEET 5F

Crossword Puzzle

Directions: Use the definitions to complete the crossword puzzles.

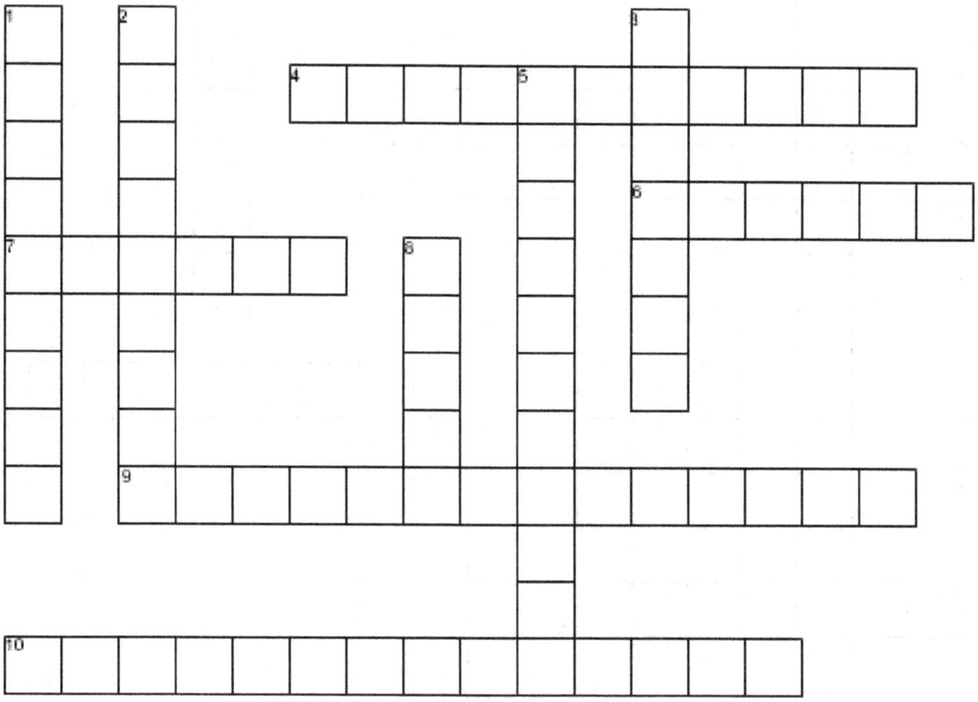

ACROSS

4 Low blood pressure

6 Heart chamber that receives blood

7 Abnormal heart sound

9 Removal of inner lining of artery

10 Also called cardioversion

DOWN

1 Electrical device to stimulate the heart

2 Pumping heart chamber

3 Area of tissue necrosis from ischemia

5 Abnormally fast heart rate

8 Stainless steel tube placed in a vessel

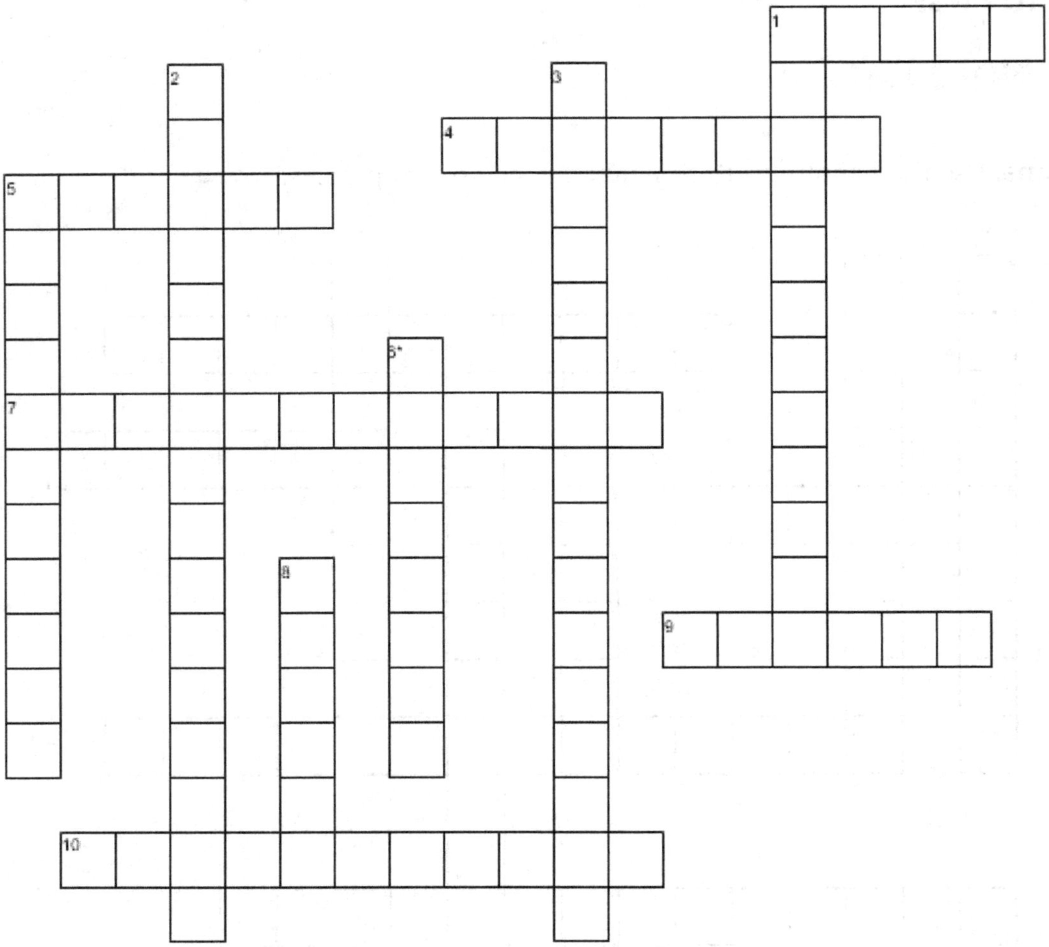

ACROSS

1 Largest artery in the body

4 ____________________ veins are swollen and distended

5 The heart is divided into halves by the ____________________

7 High blood pressure

9 Term meaning "small vein"

10 Slow heartbeat

DOWN

1 Listening to body sounds such as heart sounds

2 Term meaning "pertaining to between ventricles"

3 Term meaning "hardening of an artery"

5 Instrument used to listen to body sounds

6 Widening of the artery due to weak arterial wall

8 Blood vessel that carries blood toward the heart

WORKSHEET 5G

Chapter Review

Anatomy and Physiology

Directions: Fill in the blanks with the requested information.

1. The ________________ circulation transports deoxygenated blood to the lungs to get oxygen.
2. The ________________ is the muscular middle layer of the heart.
3. The ________________ are the upper chambers of the heart, and the ________________ are the lower pumping chambers.
4. The ________________ and ________________ valves are atrioventricular valves.
5. Another name for the mitral valve is the ________________ valve.
6. Blood ejected from the right ventricle enters the ________________, and blood ejected from the left ventricle enters the ________________.
7. The sinoatrial node is known as the ________________ of the heart.
8. ________________ are the blood vessels carrying blood away from the heart, and
9. ________________ are the blood vessels carrying blood toward the heart.
10. The narrowest blood vessels are the ________________.
11. The ________________ arteries carry blood to the heart muscle.

Word Building

Directions: Build a term for each of the following items.

1. narrowing of a vessel ________________
2. enlarged heart ________________
3. study of the heart ________________
4. surgical repair of a valve ________________
5. small vein ________________
6. pertaining to between ventricles ________________
7. heart muscle disease ________________

8. insufficient tension ______________________________

9. process of recording a vessel ______________________________

10. removal of fatty substance ______________________________

Matching

Directions: Match the term with its definition.

_____ **1.** systolic	**a.** Racing, pounding heartbeat
_____ **2.** auscultation	**b.** Thin, flexible tube inserted into body
_____ **3.** infarct	**c.** Chest pain
_____ **4.** murmur	**d.** Bacterial infection of inner layer of the heart
_____ **5.** palpitations	**e.** Congenital narrowing of aorta
_____ **6.** angina pectoris	**f.** High blood pressure
_____ **7.** cardiac arrest	**g.** Highest blood pressure reading
_____ **8.** prolapse	**h.** Portable EKG
_____ **9.** MI	**i.** Floating blood clot
_____ **10.** aneurysm	**j.** Stainless steel tube placed within vessel
_____ **11.** embolus	**k.** Varicose vein in anal region
_____ **12.** hypotension	**l.** Area of necrosis in an organ
_____ **13.** catheter	**m.** Left ventricle is too weak to pump efficiently
_____ **14.** plaque	**n.** Increases force of cardiac muscle contraction
_____ **15.** stent	**o.** Listening to body sounds
_____ **16.** regurgitation	**p.** Heart attack
_____ **17.** endocarditis	**q.** Uses radioactive thallium
_____ **18.** CoA	**r.** Loose heart valve
_____ **19.** flutter	**s.** To flow backward
_____ **20.** hemorrhoid	**t.** Also called a bruit
_____ **21.** HTN	**u.** Atria beats too fast but in regular pattern
_____ **22.** cardiac scan	**v.** Deposit of fatty lipids in an artery
_____ **23.** CHF	**w.** Localized widening of an arterial wall
_____ **24.** Holter monitor	**x.** Low blood pressure
_____ **25.** Cardiotonic	**y.** Complete stopping of heart activity

QUIZ 5A

New Word Parts

Directions: Define the combining form or suffix in the spaces provided.

1. angi/o ______________________
2. ather/o ______________________
3. cardi/o ______________________
4. atri/o ______________________
5. isch/o ______________________
6. phleb/o ______________________
7. sphygm/o ______________________
8. steth/o ______________________
9. thromb/o ______________________
10. valvul/o ______________________
11. vascul/o ______________________
12. vas/o ______________________
13. ven/o ______________________
14. ventricul/o ______________________
15. aort/o ______________________
16. arteri/o ______________________
17. coron/o ______________________
18. valv/o ______________________
19. -ule ______________________
20. -ole ______________________
21. -manometer ______________________
22. -tension ______________________
23. varic/o ______________________
24. myocardi/o ______________________

QUIZ 5B

Labeling Diagram

Directions: Label the path of blood flow through the body.

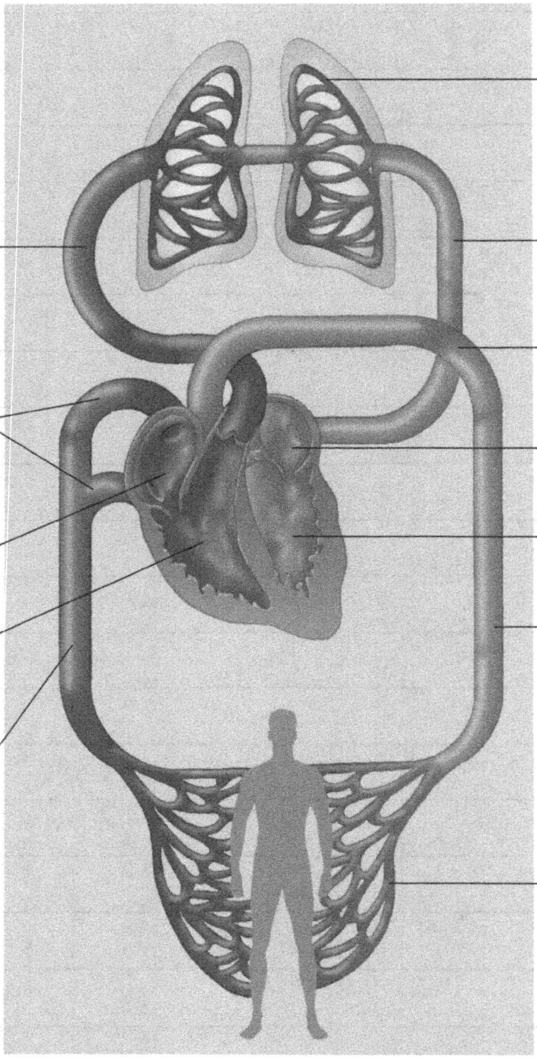

1. ______________________
2. ______________________
3. ______________________
4. ______________________
5. ______________________
6. ______________________
7. ______________________
8. ______________________
9. ______________________
10. ______________________
11. ______________________
12. ______________________

QUIZ 5C

Labeling Diagram

Directions: Label the internal structures of the heart.

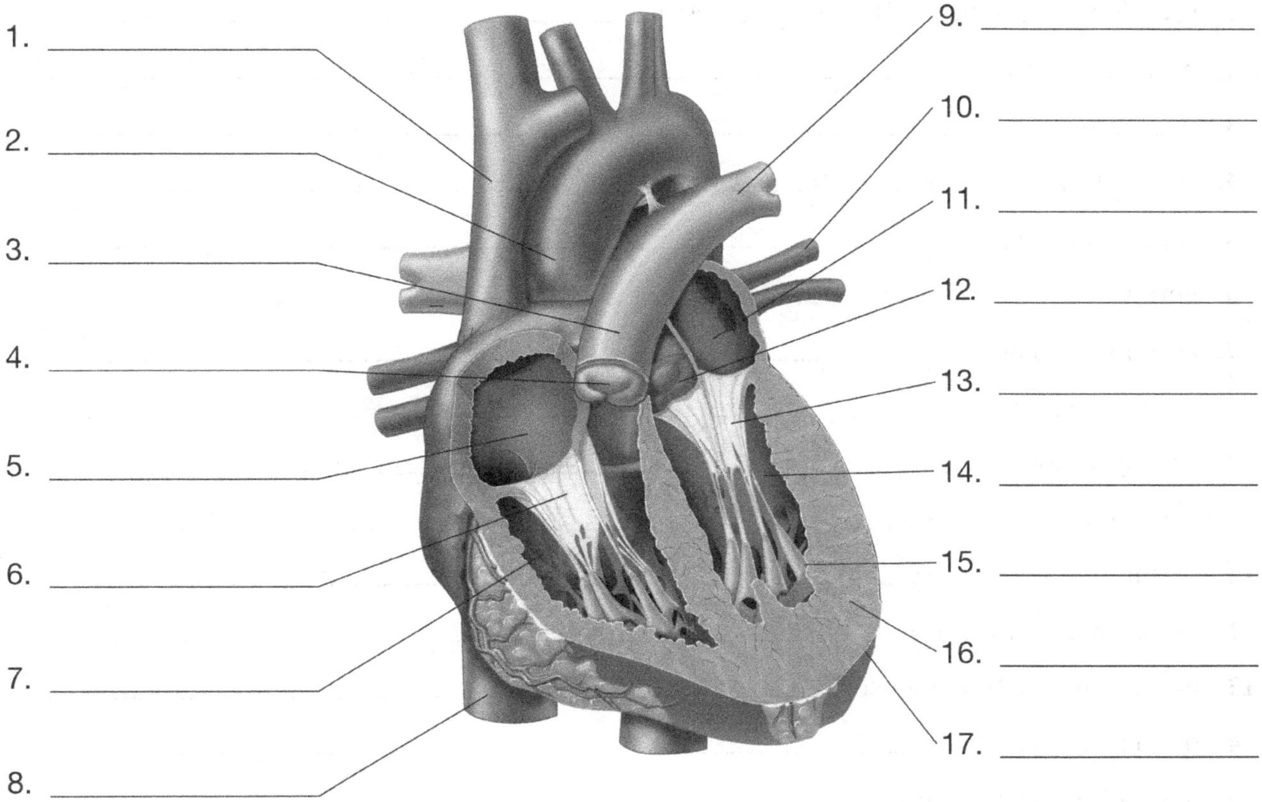

QUIZ 5D

Word Building Quiz

Directions: Build a single medical term for each phrase below.

1. involuntary muscle contraction of a vessel ______
2. narrowing of a vessel ______
3. small artery ______
4. fatty substance tumor/growth ______
5. ruptured artery ______
6. pertaining to ventricles ______
7. pertaining to atria ______
8. state of fast heart ______
9. enlarged heart ______
10. surgical repair of valve ______
11. pertaining to an artery ______
12. pertaining to the aorta ______
13. pertaining to a blood vessel ______
14. pertaining to a vein ______
15. pertaining to between ventricles ______
16. study of the heart ______
17. heart muscle disease ______
18. inflammation around heart ______
19. artery hardening ______
20. inflammation of many arteries ______
21. record of a vessel ______
22. process of recording heart electricity ______
23. pertaining to within the heart ______
24. clot destruction ______
25. pertaining to heart and lungs ______

QUIZ 5E

Abbreviations Quiz

Directions: Write the medical term for which each abbreviation stands.

1. P ______________________
2. AF ______________________
3. MI ______________________
4. BP ______________________
5. ASHD ______________________
6. CHF ______________________
7. CABG ______________________
8. CAD ______________________
9. CoA ______________________
10. CPR ______________________
11. CSD ______________________
12. HTN ______________________
13. mm Hg ______________________
14. MR ______________________
15. PDA ______________________
16. PVC ______________________
17. tPA ______________________
18. SK ______________________
19. S1 ______________________
20. MS ______________________
21. IV ______________________
22. CCU ______________________
23. CV ______________________
24. DVT ______________________
25. ECC ______________________

QUIZ 5F

Chapter Review

PART I: Multiple Choice

Directions: Circle the correct answer.

1. The pacemaker of the heart is the

a. sinoatrial node.
b. bundle of His.
c. atrioventricular node.
d. mitral valve.

2. Which circulation loop carries oxygenated blood from the heart to the cells of the body?

a. systolic
b. pulmonary
c. diastolic
d. systemic

3. Which vessel(s) bring blood to the left atrium?

a. aorta
b. pulmonary veins
c. pulmonary arteries
d. vena cavae

4. The large, thick-walled blood vessels are the

a. capillaries.
b. veins.
c. arterioles.
d. arteries.

5. The term *ischemia* is defined as

a. yellowish, fatty plaque.
b. tissue death.
c. deficiency of blood supply.
d. abnormal heart sound.

6. Abnormal quivering of heart muscle fibers is

a. palpitations.
b. murmur.
c. fibrillation.
d. angiospasm.

7. The medical term for a heart attack is

a. angina pectoris.
b. congestive heart failure.
c. arteriosclerosis.
d. myocardial infarction.

8. The congenital anomaly characterized by a connection between the pulmonary artery and the aorta is called

a. tetralogy of Fallot.
b. Raynaud's phenomenon.
c. patent ductus arteriosus.
d. congenital septal defect.

9. The surge of blood in an artery caused by the heart contraction is the
   a. pulse.
   b. blood pressure.
   c. aneurysm.
   d. pacemaker.

10. What diagnostic procedure is also known as a stress test?
   a. cardiac catheterization
   b. auscultation
   c. Holter monitor
   d. treadmill

PART II: Matching

Directions: Match the term with its definition.

____ 1. tricuspid	a. Lipid deposit in an artery
____ 2. auscultation	b. Identifies deep vein thromboses
____ 3. plaque	c. Increase indicates heart muscle damage
____ 4. thrombus	d. A heart arrhythmia
____ 5. cardiac enzymes	e. An atrioventricular heart valve
____ 6. Doppler ultrasound	f. Surgical joining of two arteries
____ 7. defibrillation	g. Blood clot forming within blood vessel
____ 8. anastomosis	h. Medication to treat hypertension
____ 9. flutter	i. Uses a stethoscope
____ 10. beta-blocker	j. Converts irregular heartbeats back to normal

PART III: Abbreviations

Directions: Write the full meaning of the following abbreviations.

1. CPR ____________________
2. ECHO ____________________
3. cath ____________________
4. CABG ____________________
5. VT ____________________

Chapter 6

Blood and the Lymphatic and Immune Systems

Learning Objectives

Upon completion of this chapter, you will be able to:

- Identify and define the combining forms and suffixes introduced in this chapter.
- Gain the ability to pronounce medical terms and major anatomical structures.
- List the major components, structures, and organs of the blood and lymphatic and immune systems and their functions.
- Describe the blood typing systems.
- Discuss immunity, the immune response, and standard precautions.
- Identify and define blood and lymphatic and immune system anatomical terms.
- Identify and define selected blood and lymphatic and immune system pathology terms.
- Identify and define selected blood and lymphatic and immune system diagnostic procedures.
- Identify and define selected blood and lymphatic and immune system therapeutic procedures.
- Identify and define selected medications associated with blood and the lymphatic and immune systems.
- Define selected abbreviations associated with blood and the lymphatic and immune systems.

WORKSHEET 6A

New Combining Form and Suffix

Directions: For each word part below, write its meaning. Then, locate a term from the chapter that uses the word part and its meaning.

Combining Forms	Meaning	Chapter Term	Meaning
1. agglutin/o			
2. bas/o			
3. chrom/o			
4. coagul/o			
5. eosin/o			
6. fibrin/o			
7. fus/o			
8. granul/o			
9. hem/o			
10. hemat/o			
11. morph/o			
12. neutr/o			
13. phag/o			
14. sanguin/o			
15. septic/o			
16. adenoid/o			
17. axill/o			
18. immun/o			
19. inguin/o			
20. lymph/o			
21. lymphaden/o			
22. lymphangi/o			
23. nucle/o			
24. splen/o			

25. thym/o ______ ______ ______

26. tonsill/o ______ ______ ______

Suffixes

27. –apheresis ______ ______ ______

28. –crit ______ ______ ______

29. –cytic ______ ______ ______

30. –cytosis ______ ______ ______

31. –emia ______ ______ ______

32. –globin ______ ______ ______

33. –penia ______ ______ ______

34. -phil ______ ______ ______

35. –philia ______ ______ ______

36. –philic ______ ______ ______

37. –plastic ______ ______ ______

38. –plastin ______ ______ ______

39. –poiesis ______ ______ ______

40. –rrhagic ______ ______ ______

41. –stasis ______ ______ ______

42. –edema ______ ______ ______

43. –globulin ______ ______ ______

44. –phage ______ ______ ______

45. –toxic ______ ______ ______

WORKSHEET 6B

Medical Term Analysis

Directions: Below are terms built from word parts used in this and previous chapters. Analyze each term presented below, and list and define the word parts used to build each term.

Medical Term	Word Part Analysis
1. basophil	______
2. eosinophil	______
3. lymphocyte	______
4. neutrophil	______
5. hemostasis	______
6. hematology	______
7. hematoma	______
8. hypochromic	______
9. morphology	______
10. phlebotomy	______
11. axillary	______
12. immunoglobulin	______
13. immunology	______
14. lymphadenitis	______
15. lymphangiography	______
16. immunotherapy	______

WORKSHEET 6C

Unscramble

Directions: Unscramble each medical term below. A definition for the term is given below each scrambled term.

1. p l a i m e o h h i ______________________________

Inherited lack of one blood-clotting factor

2. m t a m o a e h ______________________________

A bruise

3. t r m b s o i s h ______________________________

Abnormal condition of clots

4. g l u o t a e c a ______________________________

Formation of blood clot

5. l m e o n h o b i g ______________________________

Blood protein that transports oxygen

6. l a y t o p o g h ______________________________

The study of disease

7. g y l r e a l ______________________________

Hypersensitivity to common substance

8. l n m i a n f a o i t m ______________________________

Tissue response to injury

9. c a n c n i a v i o t ______________________________

Exposure to weakened pathogen to stimulate immunity

10. e l e n p s ______________________________

Organ that removes worn-out erythrocytes

WORKSHEET 6D

Sound It Out

Directions: The following are some of the important terms from this chapter written as their phonetic spellings. Sound out each term and write it in the blank.

1. an-tih-koh-AG-yoo-lant __________
2. hee-MAT-ik __________
3. an-NEE-mee-ah __________
4. hee-mah-toh-poy-EE-sis __________
5. eh-RITH-roh-sight __________
6. hee-moh-GLOH-bin __________
7. loo-KEE-mee-ah __________
8. LOO-koh-sigh-toh-sis __________
9. throm-BOH-sis __________
10. hee-moh-STAY-sis __________
11. PAN-sigh-toe-PEE-nee-ah __________
12. fleh-BOT-oh-mee __________
13. sep-tih-SEE-mee-ah __________
14. hee-moh-FILL-ee-ah __________
15. AL-er-jee __________
16. lim-fad-eh-NOP-ah-thee __________
17. im-yoo-noh-GLOB-yoo-lin __________
18. path-OL-oh-gee __________
19. in-flah-MA-shun __________
20. splen-oh-MEG-ah-lee __________
21. lim-FAN-jee-oh-gram __________
22. mon-oh-nook-lee-OH-sis __________
23. ton-sih-LEK-toh-mee __________
24. thigh-MOH-mah __________
25. ADD-eh-noy-DYE-tis __________

WORKSHEET 6E

Word Search Puzzle

Directions: Find and circle the answer for each fill-in-the-blank question in the word search puzzle.

H	H	T	E	Z	T	B	J	T	H	U
E	C	I	Q	M	Y	T	G	R	Y	R
M	T	R	V	L	B	P	X	A	J	T
O	A	C	M	H	D	O	I	G	H	I
P	R	O	T	X	D	M	L	Y	T	C
H	C	T	Z	G	E	K	M	U	V	A
I	S	A	K	K	M	U	T	Y	S	R
L	R	M	U	R	S	C	J	T	T	I
I	S	E	P	T	I	C	E	M	I	A
A	L	H	Z	Y	G	R	E	L	L	A
A	U	T	O	I	M	M	U	N	E	N

1. A(n) ______________________ is a blood test to measure the volume of red blood cells within the total volume of blood.
2. ______________________ is a cancer of leukocyte-forming red bone marrow.
3. ______________________ is commonly called blood poisoning.
4. ______________________ is commonly called a floating clot.
5. ______________________ is an inherited condition in which the blood fails to clot.
6. The ______________________ gland is an organ of the lymphatic system.
7. A(n) ______________________ is a hypersensitivity to a common substance.
8. A(n) ______________________ disease results when the body's own immune system attacks healthy cells.
9. The ______________________ test is a type of allergy testing.
10. ______________________ is the severe itching associated with hives.

WORKSHEET 6F

Crossword Puzzle

Directions: Use the definitions to complete the crossword puzzles.

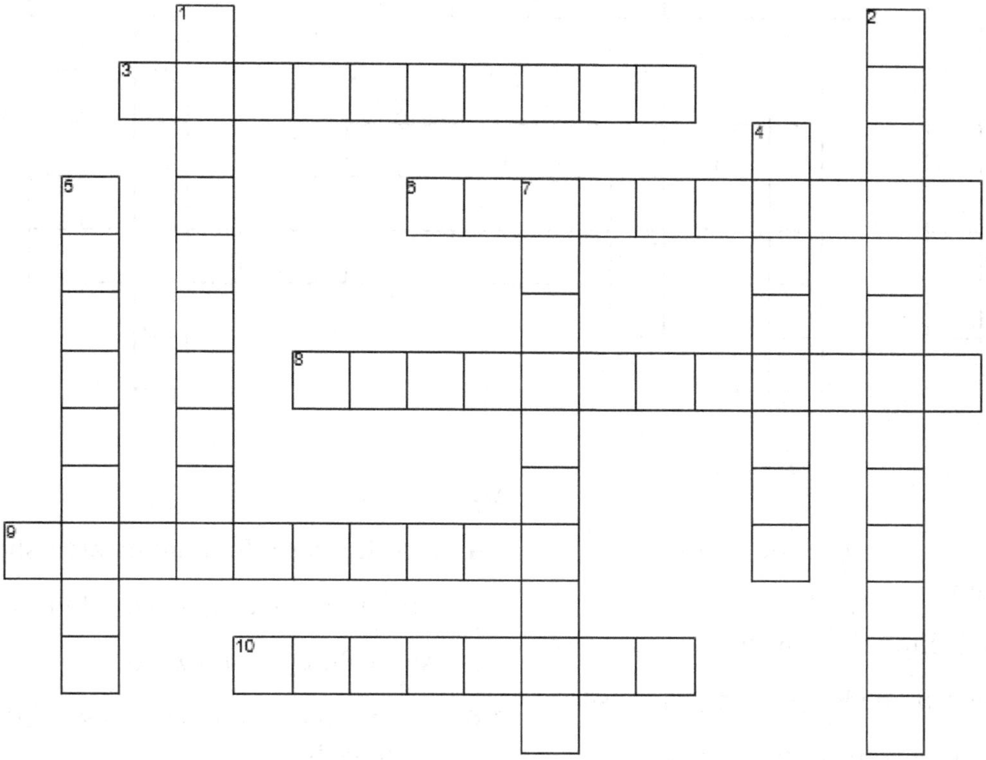

ACROSS

3 anemia results from B_{12} deficiency

6 Blood poisoning

8 Test that determines the number of each type of leukocyte

9 Test that measures the volume of red blood cells

10 Cancer of leukocyte-forming bone marrow

DOWN

1 Inherited lack of vital clotting factor

2 Substance that prevents clot formation

4 Commonly called a bruise

5 Another name for thrombocytes

7 Venipuncture

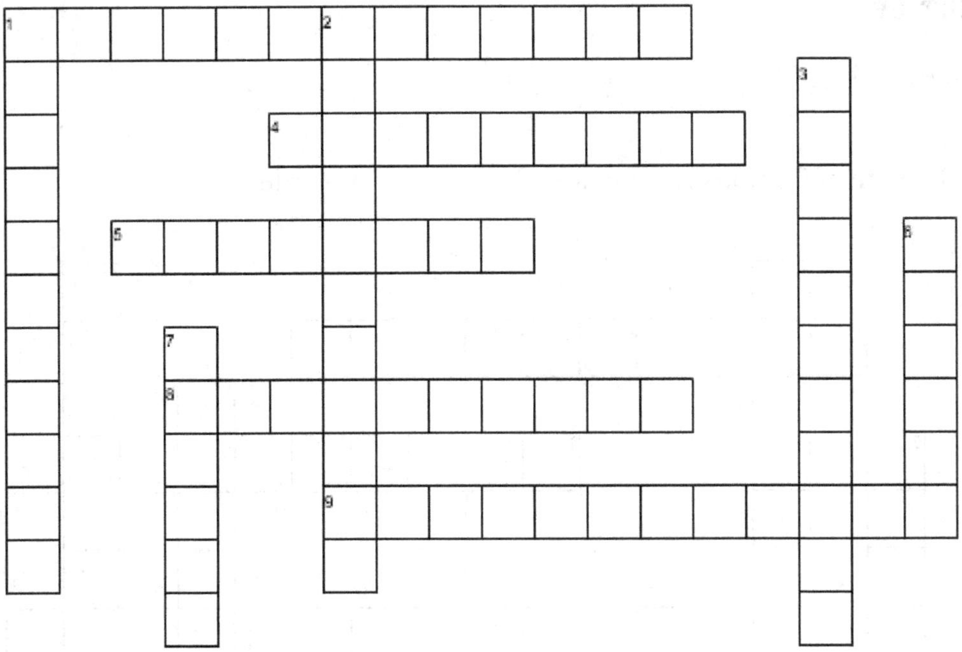

ACROSS

1 Medication to block the effects of histamine

4 Severe itching with hives

5 Common name for pharyngeal tonsils

8 Protein that transports oxygen

9 Red, painful, hot, swollen tissue response to injury

DOWN

1 Another term for anaphylactic shock

2 Autoimmune disease with fibrous lesions

3 Also called immunization

6 Organ that removes damaged red blood cells

7 Gland necessary for development of immune system

WORKSHEET 6G

Chapter Review

Anatomy and Physiology

Directions: Fill in the blanks with the requested information.

1. The formed elements of the blood are ____________________, ____________________, and ____________________.
2. The watery fluid of blood is ____________________.
3. Three examples of plasma proteins are ____________________, ____________________, and ____________________.
4. ____________________ is the iron-containing pigment that gives red blood cells their color.
5. Platelets release ____________________, which initiates the blood-clotting process.
6. The universal donor is type ____________________ blood; the universal recipient is type ______ blood.
7. ____________________ are lymphatic vessels around the small intestine.
8. Lymph nodes house ____________________ and ____________________ to remove pathogens from lymph.
9. Tonsils protect the body from invasion of pathogens through the ____________________ or ____________________ system.
10. ____________________ immunity develops following direct exposure to a pathogen.

Word Building

Directions: Build a term for each of the following items.

1. blood protein ____
2. pertaining to fibers ____
3. clotting cell ____
4. too many red cells ____
5. too few clotting (cells) ____
6. blood producing ____
7. enlarged spleen ____

8. removal of tonsils ______________________________

9. record of lymph vessels ______________________________

10. study of disease ______________________________

Matching

Directions: Match the term with its definition.

_____ **1.** allergy	**a.** Body attacks its own cells
_____ **2.** inflammation	**b.** Prevents blood-clot formation
_____ **3.** urticaria	**c.** Born with nonfunctioning immune system
_____ **4.** autoimmune disease	**d.** To stop bleeding
_____ **5.** opportunistic	**e.** Bruise
_____ **6.** anaphylaxis	**f.** Severe itching with hives
_____ **7.** Hodgkin's disease	**g.** Immunization
_____ **8.** mononucleosis	**h.** Caused by vitamin B12 deficiency
_____ **9.** SCIDS	**i.** Red bone marrow stops making blood cells
_____ **10.** vaccination	**j.** Hypersensitivity to common allergen
_____ **11.** protease inhibitor	**k.** Dissolves clots
_____ **12.** ELISA	**l.** Computer that does blood chemistry tests
_____ **13.** dyscrasia	**m.** Drug that keeps a virus from reproducing
_____ **14.** hemostasis	**n.** Cancer of lymphatic cells in lymph nodes
_____ **15.** hemophilia	**o.** Test to identify infecting bacteria
_____ **16.** aplastic anemia	**p.** Lab test for AIDS
_____ **17.** polycythemia vera	**q.** Infection occurring in immunocompromised
_____ **18.** C&S	**r.** Measures volume of erythrocytes in blood
_____ **19.** phlebotomy	**s.** General term for blood condition
_____ **20.** anticoagulant	**t.** Tissues' response to injury
_____ **21.** thrombolytic	**u.** Venipuncture
_____ **22.** SMAC	**v.** Prolonged blood-clotting time
_____ **23.** hematocrit	**w.** Life-threatening allergic reaction
_____ **24.** pernicious anemia	**x.** Too many red blood cells
_____ **25.** hematoma	**y.** Caused by Epstein-Barr virus

QUIZ 6A

New Word Parts Quiz

Directions: Define the combining form or suffix in the spaces provided.

1. thromb/o ______
2. agglutin/o ______
3. chrom/o ______
4. coagul/o ______
5. erythr/o ______
6. fibrin/o ______
7. hemat/o ______
8. phag/o ______
9. leuk/o ______
10. morph/o ______
11. sanguin/o ______
12. eosin/o ______
13. thym/o ______
14. adenoid/o ______
15. tonsill/o ______
16. tox/o ______
17. splen/o ______
18. lymphaden/o ______
19. lymphangi/o ______
20. -cytosis ______
21. -globin ______
22. -poiesis ______
23. -penia ______
24. -stasis ______

QUIZ 6B

Labeling Diagram

Directions: Label the components of whole blood.

1. ______________________

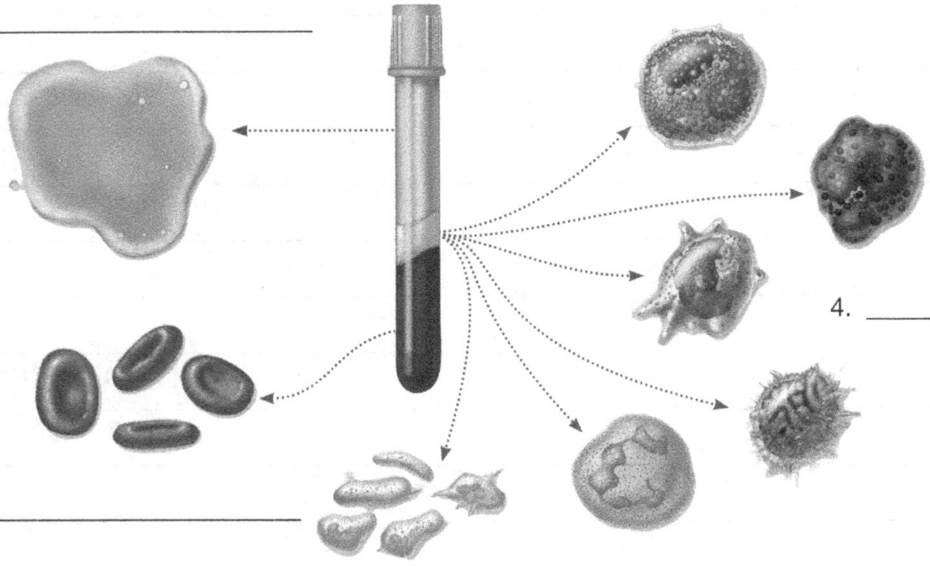

4. ______________________

2. ______________________

3. ______________________

QUIZ 6C

Labeling Diagram

Directions: Label the organs of the lymphatic system.

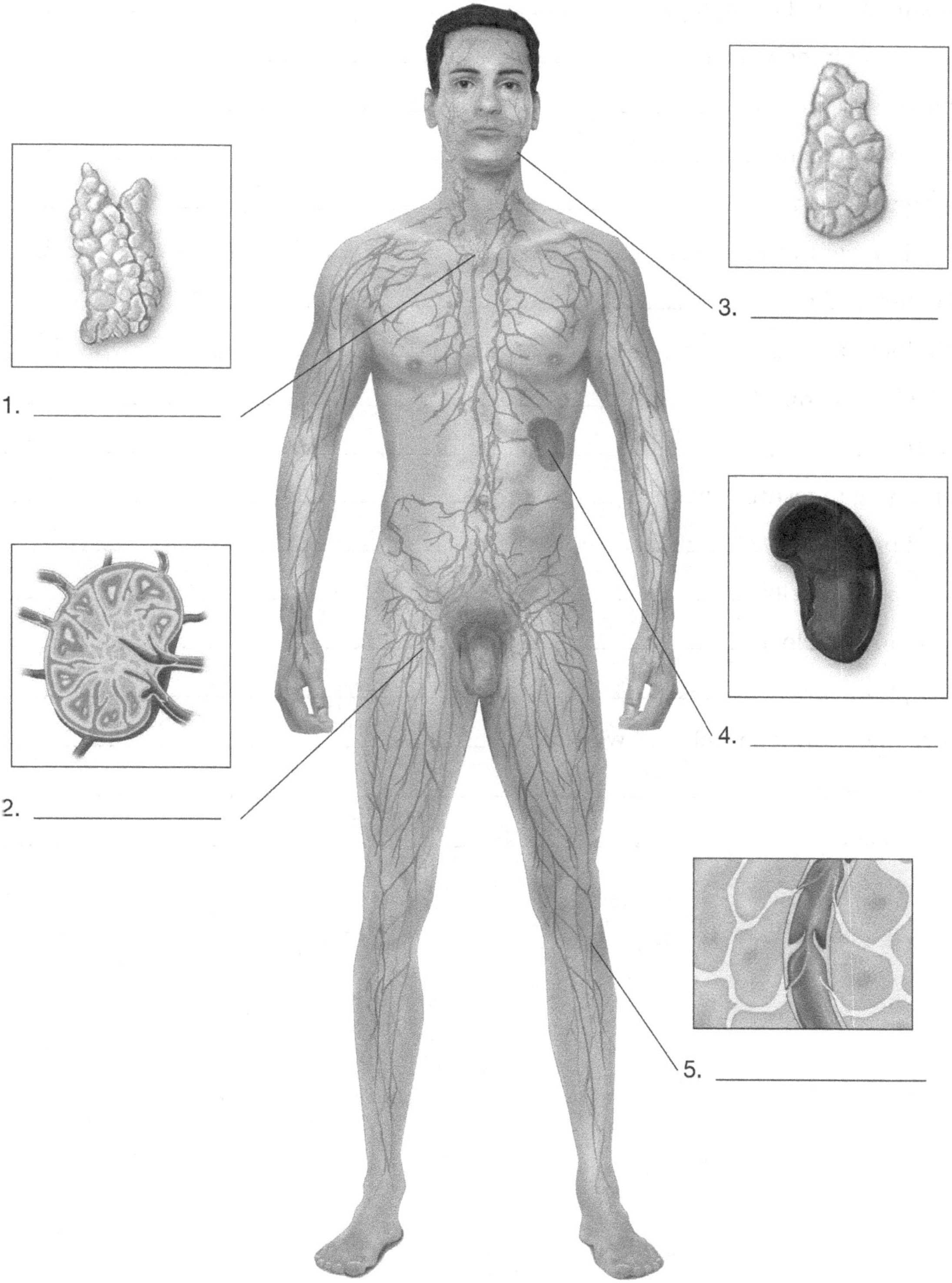

QUIZ 6D

Word Building Quiz

Directions: Build a single medical term for each phrase below.

1. inflammation of adenoids ______
2. removal of lymph gland ______
3. lymph vessel tumor ______
4. disease producing ______
5. enlarged spleen ______
6. pertaining to tonsils ______
7. clot dissolving ______
8. vein incision ______
9. cell without granules ______
10. red cell ______
11. pertaining to insufficient color ______
12. blood protein ______
13. too few of all cells ______
14. rapid flow of blood ______
15. fiber producing ______
16. more than normal number of white cells ______
17. blood stopping ______
18. blood mass ______

QUIZ 6E

Abbreviations Quiz

Directions: Write the medical term for which each abbreviation stands.

1. AIDS ____________________
2. GVHD ____________________
3. HD ____________________
4. Ig ____________________
5. mono ____________________
6. KS ____________________
7. NK ____________________
8. PCP ____________________
9. SCIDS ____________________
10. HIV ____________________
11. CBC ____________________
12. BMT ____________________
13. diff ____________________
14. ESR ____________________
15. ECT ____________________
16. Hgb ____________________
17. PA ____________________
18. PT ____________________
19. RBC ____________________
20. WBC ____________________
21. SMAC ____________________
22. lymphs ____________________
23. ALL ____________________
24. eosins ____________________
25. monos ____________________

QUIZ 6F

Chapter Review

PART I: Multiple Choice

Directions: Circle the correct answer.

1. blood disorder characterized by excessive increase in abnormal white blood cells is
   - **a.** Hodgkin's disease.
   - **b.** leukemia.
   - **c.** hemophilia.
   - **d.** leukopenia.
2. The lymph nodes located in the underarm region are termed
   - **a.** axillary.
   - **b.** cervical.
   - **c.** mediastinal.
   - **d.** inguinal.
3. Which blood type is known as the universal recipient?
   - **a.** type O
   - **b.** type A
   - **c.** type B
   - **d.** type AB
4. An example of active acquired immunity is
   - **a.** mother's antibodies crossing placenta.
   - **b.** having the disease.
   - **c.** receiving an antitoxin.
   - **d.** macrophages engulfing bacteria.
5. Which is *not* a type of leukocyte?
   - **a.** basophil
   - **b.** eosinophil
   - **c.** thrombin
   - **d.** lymphocyte
6. Which blood test measures the volume of erythrocytes in a given volume of blood?
   - **a.** differential
   - **b.** bleeding time
   - **c.** hematocrit
   - **d.** hemoglobin
7. Which is a test for infectious mononucleosis?
   - **a.** white cell differential
   - **b.** prothrombin time
   - **c.** erythrocyte sedimentation rate
   - **d.** monospot
8. In which type of blood transfusion does the blood come from another person?
   - **a.** packed red cells
   - **b.** dialysis transfusion
   - **c.** autologous transfusion
   - **d.** homologous transfusion

9. The largest lymph vessels are called
   - a. ducts.
   - b. arteries.
   - c. capillaries.
   - d. valves.

10. Which type of anemia is inherited?
    - a. pernicious anemia
    - b. aplastic anemia
    - c. sickle cell anemia
    - d. iron-deficiency anemia

PART II: Matching

Directions: Match the term with its definition.

_____ 1. platelets	a. Increases number of erythrocytes
_____ 2. ABO	b. Plasma and formed elements
_____ 3. whole blood	c. Pharyngeal tonsils
_____ 4. septicemia	d. Test for inflammation in the body
_____ 5. sed rate	e. Acquired in a hospital
_____ 6. hematinic	f. Play role in blood-clotting process
_____ 7. adenoids	g. Caused by blocked lymph flow
_____ 8. nosocomial infection	h. An autoimmune disease
_____ 9. lymphedema	i. Blood poisoning
_____ 10. sarcoidosis	j. Blood typing system

PART III: Abbreviations

Directions: Write the full meaning of the following abbreviations.

1. ARC ______________________________
2. GVHD ______________________________
3. PCP ______________________________
4. CBC ______________________________
5. PA ______________________________

Chapter 7

Respiratory System

Learning Objectives

Upon completion of this chapter, you will be able to:

- Identify and define the combining forms and suffixes introduced in this chapter.
- Correctly spell and pronounce medical terms and major anatomical structures relating to the respiratory system.
- Locate and describe the major organs of the respiratory system and their functions.
- List and describe the lung volumes and capacities.
- Describe the process of respiration.
- Identify and define respiratory system anatomical terms.
- Identify and define selected respiratory system pathology terms.
- Identify and define selected respiratory system diagnostic procedures.
- Identify and define selected respiratory system therapeutic procedures.
- Identify and define selected medications relating to the respiratory system.
- Define selected abbreviations associated with the respiratory system.

WORKSHEET 7A

New Combining Form and Suffix

Directions: For each word part below, write its meaning. Then, locate a term from the chapter that uses the word part and its meaning.

Combining Forms	Meaning	Chapter Term	Meaning
1. aer/o			
2. alveol/o			
3. anthrac/o			
4. atel/o			
5. bronch/o			
6. bronchi/o			
7. bronchiol/o			
8. coni/o			
9. cyano/o			
10. cyst/o			
11. diaphragmat/o			
12. epiglott/o			
13. hal/o			
14. laryng/o			
15. lob/o			
16. muc/o			
17. nas/o			
18. ox/o, ox/i			
19. pharyng/o			
20. pleur/o			
21. pneum/o			
22. pneumon/o			
23. pulmon/o			
24. rhin/o			

25. sept/o ______ ______ ______

26. sinus/o ______ ______ ______

27. somn/o ______ ______ ______

28. spir/o ______ ______ ______

29. trache/o ______ ______ ______

30. tuss/o ______ ______ ______

Suffixes

31. -capnia ______ ______ ______

32. -osmia ______ ______ ______

33. -phonia ______ ______ ______

34. -pnea ______ ______ ______

35. -ptysis ______ ______ ______

36. -thorax ______ ______ ______

WORKSHEET 7B

Medical Term Analysis

Directions: Below are terms built from word parts used in this and previous chapters. Analyze each term presented below, and list and define the word parts used to build each term.

Medical Term	Word Part Analysis
1. paranasal	______
2. alveolar	______
3. nasopharyngitis	______
4. visceral	______
5. cyanosis	______
6. hemoptysis	______
7. otorhinolaryngology	______
8. fibrosis	______
9. atelectasis	______
10. pneumoconiosis	______
11. cytology	______
12. bronchography	______
13. bronchoscopy	______
14. angiography	______
15. laryngoscopy	______
16. oximetry	______
17. spirometry	______
18. tracheotomy	______
19. thoracocentesis	______
20. cardiopulmonary	______

WORKSHEET 7C

Unscramble

Directions: Unscramble each medical term below. A definition for the term is given below each scrambled term.

1. h p y s m m a e e ______________________

   Condition resulting from the destruction of alveolar walls

2. p m b c r h n s s a o o ______________________

   Involuntary muscle spasm in a bronchus

3. n a l f u n i z e ______________________

   Viral infection with chills, fever, body aches, and dry cough

4. n i n m e u p o a ______________________

   Death may occur as alveoli fill up with fluid

5. r e o n i t v a t l ______________________

   Mechanical device that assists in breathing

6. s c o a s i n y ______________________

   Abnormal condition of being blue

7. p r a y l g o s n c e o ______________________

   Instrument to view the voice box

8. s p e i t a s i x ______________________

   Nosebleed

9. h i n s r l p a o y t ______________________

   Surgical repair of the nose

10. a o s n h r p a n e g a l y ______________________

    Pertaining to the nose and throat

WORKSHEET 7D

Sound It Out

Directions: The following are some of the important terms from this chapter written as their phonetic spellings. Sound out each term and write it in the blank.

1. AP-nee-ah ______
2. AZ-mah ______
3. al-vee-OH-lar ______
4. sigh-ah-NO-sis ______
5. em-fih-SEE-mah ______
6. PULL-mon-air-ee ______
7. in-floo-EN-za ______
8. en-doh-TRAY-kee-al ______
9. brong-KOG-rah-fee ______
10. new-moh-THOH-raks ______
11. too-ber-kyoo-LOH-sis ______
12. tho-RASS-ik ______
13. spy-ROM-eh-tree ______
14. ploor-oh-sen-TEE-sis ______
15. ah-NOK-see-ah ______
16. thor-ah-KOT-oh-mee ______
17. ah-NOZ-mee-ah ______
18. dif-THEAR-ee-ah ______
19. dis-FOH-nee-ah ______
20. lair-RING-go-scope ______
21. pan-sigh-nus-EYE-tis ______
22. per-TUH-is ______
23. rye-NYE-tis ______
24. rye-noh-REE-ah ______
25. tray-kee-oh-steh-NOH-sis ______

WORKSHEET 7E

Word Search Puzzle

Directions: Find and circle the answer for each fill-in-the-blank question in the word search puzzle.

H	Y	P	E	R	V	E	N	T	I	L	A	T	I	O	N
F	V	H	F	B	B	R	H	V	R	L	F	T	Q	N	N
Q	T	T	R	S	I	S	S	U	T	R	E	P	J	P	J
Z	N	T	J	T	N	S	N	B	T	M	M	Q	M	H	M
V	G	B	G	R	Y	K	I	D	X	R	Y	L	K	D	P
S	L	Z	X	Y	B	P	A	X	T	J	R	K	E	T	N
V	P	M	B	T	H	U	I	W	A	P	Z	C	Z	W	E
W	L	U	L	P	Z	O	X	N	R	T	O	Q	K	N	U
Y	Z	T	T	N	P	R	Y	Q	M	N	S	A	D	K	M
J	C	T	Y	U	R	C	H	Z	G	G	L	I	K	K	O
R	W	V	O	L	M	N	P	E	K	U	B	G	P	R	T
Z	M	R	B	M	P	N	S	K	N	K	M	G	R	E	H
F	C	F	C	P	C	T	A	N	K	L	L	J	P	H	O
Z	K	C	L	H	A	L	A	P	K	T	D	N	M	N	R
T	T	K	L	N	Z	C	T	P	K	K	L	H	K	F	A
R	Y	R	T	P	Q	F	L	C	J	J	V	G	L	X	X

1. ______________________________ is also called suffocation.
2. ______________ is a viral infection in children with a characteristic barking cough.
3. Breathing too fast and too deep is called ______________________________.
4. When phlegm is coughed up and expelled through the mouth, it is called __________.
5. ______________________________ may result in a collapsed lung.
6. A(n) ____________________ is a medication to reduce nasal and sinus stuffiness.
7. The medical term for whooping cough is ______________________________.
8. ______________________________ is the medical term for nosebleed.
9. The symptoms of ____________________ include a barking cough.
10. A nasal ________________ is a two-pronged plastic device for delivering oxygen.

WORKSHEET 7F

Crossword Puzzle

Directions: Use the definitions to complete the crossword puzzles.

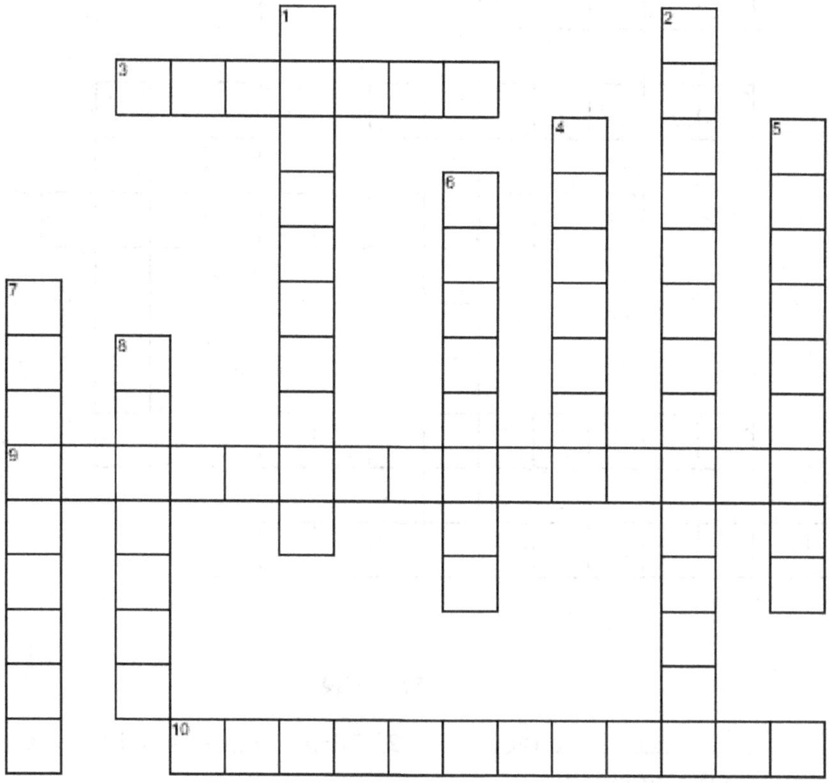

ACROSS

3 Term meaning "difficulty breathing"

9 Breathing too slowly and too shallowly

10 Results in the collapse of a lung

DOWN

1 Instrument to measure breathing

2 Medication that widens bronchi

4 Commonly called windpipe

5 Infection in which fluid fills the alveoli

6 Inflammation of pleura

7 Condition that destroys alveolar walls

8 Term for insufficient oxygen in the body

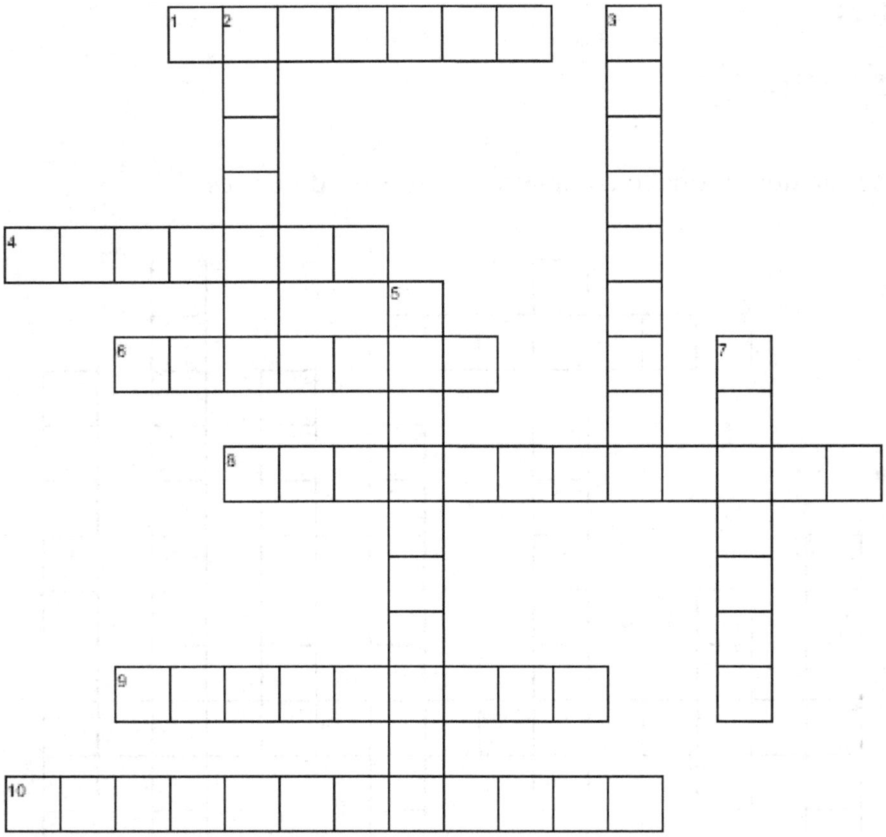

ACROSS

1 A nasal ____________________ delivers oxygen directly into the nose

4 Term meaning "without carbon dioxide"

6 Anatomical name for windpipe

8 Medication to reduce nasal stuffiness

9 Whooping cough

10 Term meaning "process of viewing voice box"

DOWN

2 Term meaning "without voice"

3 Nosebleed

5 Term meaning "spitting up blood"

7 Anatomical name for throat

WORKSHEET 7G

Chapter Review

Anatomy and Physiology

Directions: Fill in the blanks with the requested information.

1. The three parts of respiration are ____________________, ____________________, and ____________________.
2. Inhalation brings in fresh ____________________ and exhalation removes ____________________ from the body.
3. The nasal cavity and much of the respiratory tract is covered by ____________________, which secretes a sticky fluid called ____________________.
4. The eustachian tube extends from the ____________________ to the ____________________.
5. The ____________________ is a flap of cartilage that covers the larynx to prevent food from entering the trachea.
6. The smallest bronchial tubes are called ____________________.
7. ____________________ are the air sacs in the lungs.
8. The bronchi, pulmonary blood vessels, and nerves enter each lung along its medial border in an area called the ____________________.
9. ____________________ is the volume of air that moves into or out of your lungs during quiet breathing.
10. The vital signs consist of ____________________, ____________________, ____________________, and ____________________.

Word Building

Directions: Build a term for each of the following items.

1. surgical repair of bronchus ______________________________
2. inflammation of voice box ______________________________
3. removal of lobe ______________________________
4. condition of no oxygen ______________________________
5. puncture pleura to withdraw fluid ______________________________
6. nose discharge ______________________________
7. inflammation of all sinuses ______________________________
8. pertaining to throat ______________________________
9. blood in chest ______________________________
10. fast breathing ______________________________

Matching

Directions: Match the term with its definition.

____ **1.** epistaxis
____ **2.** cyanosis
____ **3.** hyperventilation
____ **4.** nasal cannula
____ **5.** hemoptysis
____ **6.** patent
____ **7.** crackles
____ **8.** SOB
____ **9.** rhonchi
____ **10.** pertussis
____ **11.** stridor
____ **12.** anthracosis
____ **13.** CF
____ **14.** emphysema
____ **15.** histoplasmosis
____ **16.** MDI
____ **17.** empyema
____ **18.** SIDS
____ **19.** ABGs
____ **20.** sputum cytology
____ **21.** laryngoscopy
____ **22.** polysomnography
____ **23.** ventilator
____ **24.** antitussive
____ **25.** expectorant

a. Coughing up blood
b. Wheezing sound
c. A blood test
d. Dyspnea
e. Test for sleep apnea
f. Harsh, high-pitched breath sound
g. Improves ability to cough up mucus
h. Two-pronged plastic device to deliver oxygen
i. Inherited condition
j. Pyothorax
k. Nosebleed
l. Destruction of alveolar walls
m. Metered-dose inhaler
n. Test looking for malignant cells
o. Breathe too fast and too deep
p. Visual examination of voice box
q. Crackling sound
r. Respirator
s. Whooping cough
t. Open
u. Reduces urge to cough
v. Black lung
w. Unexplained death of apparently well infant
x. Fungal infection
y. Bluish tint to skin

QUIZ 7A

New Word Parts Quiz

Directions: Define the combining form or suffix in the spaces provided.

1. bronchiol/o ______________________________

2. atel/o ______________________________

3. coni/o ______________________________

4. epiglott/o ______________________________

5. laryng/o ______________________________

6. pharyng/o ______________________________

7. trache/o ______________________________

8. pulmon/o ______________________________

9. pneum/o ______________________________

10. ox/i ______________________________

11. cyan/o ______________________________

12. nas/o ______________________________

13. anthrac/o ______________________________

14. pleur/o ______________________________

15. sinus/o ______________________________

16. spir/o ______________________________

17. rhin/o ______________________________

18. alveol/o ______________________________

19. bronchi/o ______________________________

20. diaphragmat/o ______________________________

21. -capnia ______________________________

22. -thorax ______________________________

23. -osmia ______________________________

24. -pnea ______________________________

25. –ptysis ______________________________

QUIZ 7B

Labeling Diagram

Directions: Label the structures of the upper respiratory system.

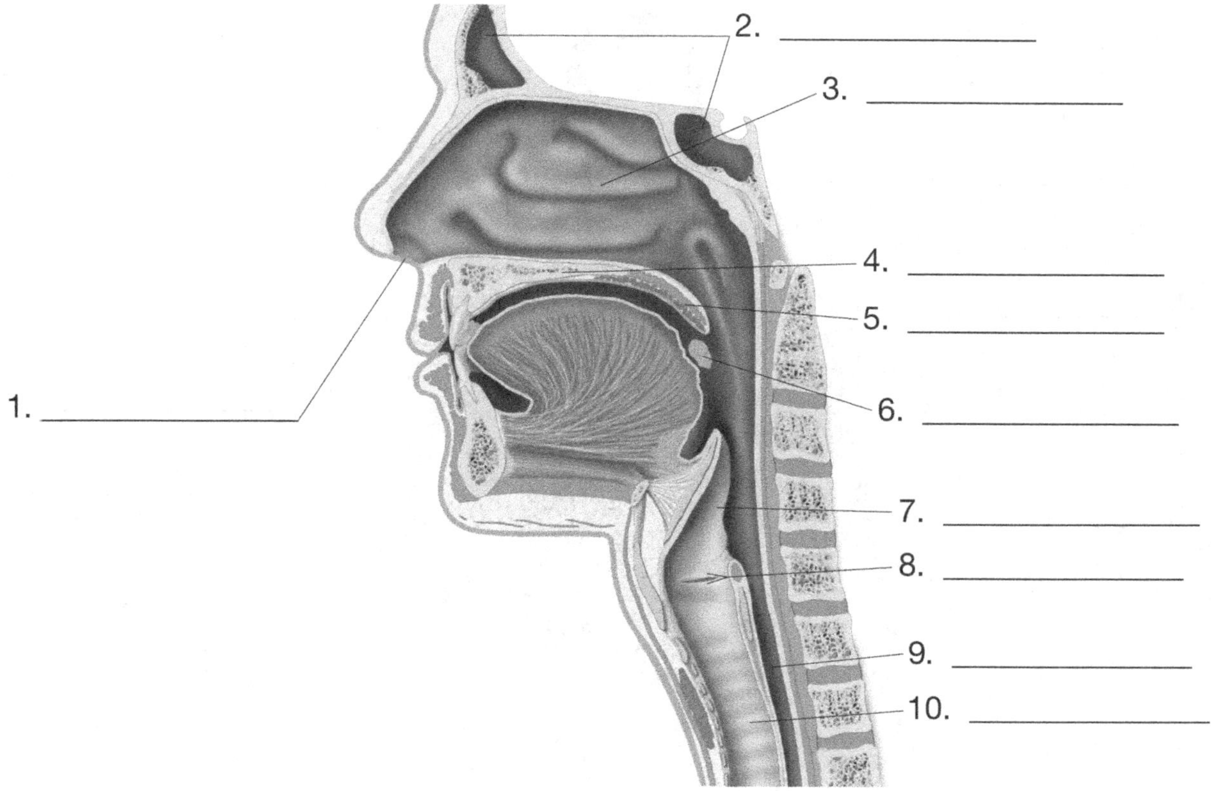

QUIZ 7C

Labeling Diagram

Directions: Label the structures of the lungs.

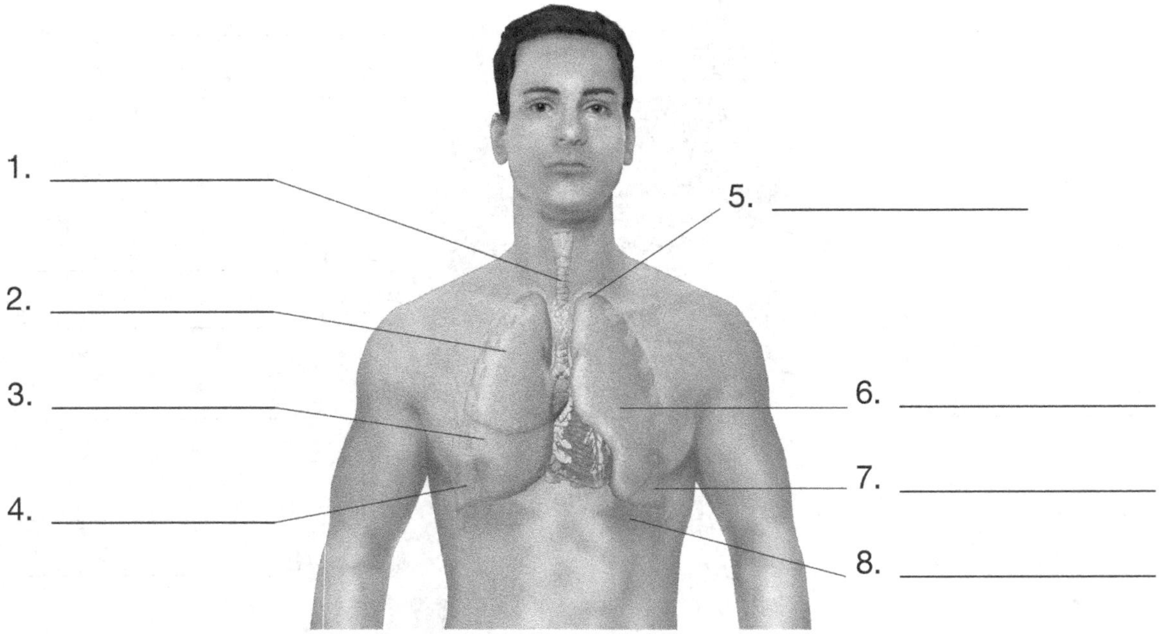

QUIZ 7D

Word Building Quiz

Directions: Build a single medical term for each phrase below.

1. surgical repair of bronchus ______
2. instrument to view inside bronchus ______
3. removal of voice box ______
4. paralysis of voice box ______
5. puncture of pleura to withdraw fluid ______
6. condition of insufficient oxygen ______
7. lung specialist ______
8. nose discharge ______
9. abnormal condition of nose fungus ______
10. instrument to measure oxygen ______
11. removal of lobe ______
12. chest pain ______
13. inflammation of all sinuses ______
14. inflammation of nose and throat ______
15. pleural pain ______
16. pertaining to lung ______
17. pertaining to inside trachea ______
18. pertaining to chest ______
19. pertaining to voice box ______
20. no voice ______
21. excessive carbon dioxide ______
22. no smell ______
23. slow breathing ______
24. pus in chest ______
25. normal breathing ______

QUIZ 7E

Abbreviations Quiz

Directions: Write the medical term for which each abbreviation stands.

1. ABGs ____________________
2. ARDS ____________________
3. CO2 ____________________
4. COPD ____________________
5. CTA ____________________
6. CXR ____________________
7. ENT ____________________
8. IPPB ____________________
9. IRDS ____________________
10. LLL ____________________
11. MDI ____________________
12. O2 ____________________
13. PFT ____________________
14. RA ____________________
15. RDS ____________________
16. RRT ____________________
17. SARS ____________________
18. SIDS ____________________
19. SOB ____________________
20. TB ____________________
21. TLC ____________________
22. TPR ____________________
23. TV ____________________
24. URI ____________________
25. CPR ____________________

QUIZ 7F

Chapter Review

PART I: Multiple Choice

Directions: Circle the correct answer.

1. The volume of air that can be exhaled after a maximum inhalation is
   - **a.** inspiratory reserve volume.
   - **b.** tidal volume.
   - **c.** total lung volume.
   - **d.** vital capacity.
2. The term for abnormal "crackling" sounds made during inspiration is
   - **a.** pleural rub.
   - **b.** rales.
   - **c.** rhonchi.
   - **d.** stridor.
3. The acute respiratory condition found in infants characterized by a barking cough is
   - **a.** asthma.
   - **b.** bronchitis.
   - **c.** croup.
   - **d.** laryngitis.
4. The name for the condition in which an area of lung tissue collapses is
   - **a.** bronchiectasis.
   - **b.** atelectasis.
   - **c.** emphysema.
   - **d.** asthma.
5. When lung tissue retains an excessive amount of fluid, this is called
   - **a.** pulmonary edema.
   - **b.** pulmonary embolism.
   - **c.** pleural effusion.
   - **d.** thoracalgia.
6. The medical term that means open or unblocked is
   - **a.** aspirate.
   - **b.** asphyxia.
   - **c.** patent.
   - **d.** rhonchi.
7. Which abbreviation stands for an acute respiratory syndrome?
   - **a.** SARS
   - **b.** TPR
   - **c.** PFT
   - **d.** ARDS
8. A laboratory test for the presence of malignant cells is
   - **a.** sputum culture and sensitivity.
   - **b.** throat culture.
   - **c.** endotracheal intubation.
   - **d.** sputum cytology.

9. The term for using a device to measure the breathing capacity of the lungs is
   - **a.** pulmonary angiography.
   - **b.** intermittent positive pressure breathing.
   - **c.** spirometry.
   - **d.** bronchography.

10. Using the fingertips to tap on a surface to determine the condition beneath is called
   - **a.** auscultation.
   - **b.** palpation.
   - **c.** inspection.
   - **d.** percussion.

PART II: Matching

Directions: Match the term with its definition.

_____ **1.** nares	**a.** Normal breathing
_____ **2.** glottis	**b.** May cause severe bronchospasms
_____ **3.** eupnea	**c.** A type of pneumoconiosis
_____ **4.** aspiration	**d.** External openings of the nose
_____ **5.** phlegm	**e.** Causes walking pneumonia
_____ **6.** asthma	**f.** A nuclear medicine test
_____ **7.** *Mycoplasma*	**g.** Thick mucus of the respiratory tract
_____ **8.** silicosis	**h.** Opening through vocal cords
_____ **9.** ventilation-perfusion scan	**i.** Blocks allergy attack
_____ **10.** antihistamine	**j.** Withdraws fluid using suction

PART III: Abbreviations

Directions: Write the full meaning of the following abbreviations.

1. COPD ______________________________
2. TPR ______________________________
3. URI ______________________________
4. SOB ______________________________
5. CXR ______________________________

Chapter 8

Digestive System

Learning Objectives

Upon completion of this chapter, you will be able to:

- Identify and define the combining forms and suffixes introduced in this chapter.
- Correctly spell and pronounce medical terms and major anatomical structures relating to the digestive system.
- Locate and describe the major organs of the digestive system and their functions.
- Identify the shape and function of each type of tooth.
- Describe the function of the accessory organs of the digestive system.
- Identify and define digestive system anatomical terms.
- Identify and define selected digestive system pathology terms.
- Identify and define selected digestive system diagnostic procedures.
- Identify and define selected digestive system therapeutic procedures.
- Identify and define selected medications relating to the digestive system.
- Define selected abbreviations associated with the digestive system.

WORKSHEET 8A

New Combining Form and Suffix

Directions: For each word part below, write its meaning. Then, locate a term from the chapter that uses the word part and its meaning.

Combining Forms	Meaning	Chapter Term	Meaning
1. an/o			
2. append/o			
3. appendic/o			
4. bar/o			
5. bucc/o			
6. cec/o			
7. cholangi/o			
8. chol/e			
9. cholecyst/o			
10. choledoch/o			
11. cirrh/o			
12. col/o			
13. colon/o			
14. dent/o			
15. diverticul/o			
16. duoden/o			
17. enter/o			
18. esophag/o			
19. gastr/o			
20. gingiv/o			
21. gloss/o			
22. hepat/o			
23. ile/o			
24. jejun/o			

25. labi/o ______ ______ ______
26. lapar/o ______ ______ ______
27. lingu/o ______ ______ ______
28. lith/o ______ ______ ______
29. odont/o ______ ______ ______
30. or/o ______ ______ ______
31. palat/o ______ ______ ______
32. pancreat/o ______ ______ ______
33. pharyng/o ______ ______ ______
34. polyp/o ______ ______ ______
35. proct/o ______ ______ ______
36. pylor/o ______ ______ ______
37. pyr/o ______ ______ ______
38. rect/o ______ ______ ______
39. sialaden/o ______ ______ ______
40. sigmoid/o ______ ______ ______

Suffixes

41. –emesis ______ ______ ______
42. –emetic ______ ______ ______
43. –iatric ______ ______ ______
44. –istry ______ ______ ______
45. –lithiasis ______ ______ ______
46. –orexia ______ ______ ______
47. –pepsia ______ ______ ______
48. –phagia ______ ______ ______
49. –prandial ______ ______ ______
50. –tripsy ______ ______ ______

WORKSHEET 8B

Medical Term Analysis

Directions: Below are terms built from word parts used in this and previous chapters. Analyze each term presented below, and list and define the word parts used to build each term.

Medical Term	Word Part Analysis
1. proctology	______________________
2. gastroesophageal	______________________
3. carcinoma	______________________
4. colitis	______________________
5. cholecystitis	______________________
6. cholelithiasis	______________________
7. cholecystography	______________________
8. intravenous	______________________
9. transhepatic	______________________
10. cholangiography	______________________
11. colonoscopy	______________________
12. cholangiopancreatography	______________________
13. esophagogastroduodenoscopy	______________________
14. gastroscopy	______________________
15. laparoscopy	______________________
16. sigmoidoscopy	______________________
17. choledocholithotripsy	______________________

WORKSHEET 8C

Unscramble

Directions: Unscramble each medical term below. A definition for the term is given below each scrambled term.

1. i s d a a n e i t s i l ____________________

   Inflammation of a salivary gland

2. l v s u l v u o ____________________

   Bowel twists upon itself

3. c p t o o o y r g l ____________________

   Medical specialty in the study of the rectum and anus

4. h r i c r o i s s ____________________

   Chronic liver disease

5. o m r s h i r h d e o ____________________

   Varicose veins in the rectum

6. n t s e d y e y r ____________________

   Condition with pain, diarrhea, and blood and mucus in the stool

7. s a t g o n e r r e i t i s t ____________________

   Inflammation of stomach and small intestines

8. m s e a h m e s e t i ____________________

   Vomiting blood

9. a i n e d j c u ____________________

   Yellow skin color associated with liver disease

10. t n c a i t m e e i ____________________

    Medication to treat nausea and vomiting

WORKSHEET 8D

Sound It Out

Directions: The following are some of the important terms from this chapter written as their phonetic spellings. Sound out each term and write it in the blank.

1. sig-MOYD-oh-scope ______________________
2. gas-TRY-tis ______________________
3. sih-ROH-sis ______________________
4. koh-lon-OSS-koh-pee ______________________
5. kohl-oh-REK-tall ______________________
6. koh-lee-sis-TEK-toh-mee ______________________
7. dis-PEP-see-ah ______________________
8. ah-FAY-jee-ah ______________________
9. en-TARE-ik ______________________
10. gas-troh-en-ter-EYE-tis ______________________
11. JAWN-diss ______________________
12. hee-mah-TEM-eh-sis ______________________
13. ah-pen-dih-SIGH-tis ______________________
14. HEM-oh-roydz ______________________
15. dis-in-TARE-ee ______________________
16. high-per-EM-eh-sis ______________________
17. ill-ee-OSS-toh-mee ______________________
18. jih-JUNE-all ______________________
19. lap-ar-OSS-koh-pee ______________________
20. me-LEE-nah ______________________
21. pan-kree-AT-ik ______________________
22. dis-FAY-jee-ah ______________________
23. gas-TREK-toh-mee ______________________
24. hep-AT-ik ______________________
25. VOL-vyoo-lus ______________________

WORKSHEET 8E

Word Search Puzzle

Directions: Find and circle the answer for each fill-in-the-blank question in the word search puzzle.

N	V	X	F	H	E	M	O	R	R	H	O	I	D	S
S	J	X	K	B	P	M	X	K	S	L	L	N	I	J
P	E	W	T	N	T	N	W	E	J	J	J	T	X	K
N	V	T	K	R	A	Z	C	Y	S	T	I	U	M	D
L	Z	J	I	U	W	I	C	X	I	T	Z	S	J	C
E	F	N	S	C	R	L	C	Y	S	R	V	S	K	Y
C	M	E	X	A	S	Z	R	Y	O	J	M	U	N	M
I	A	E	V	R	R	A	C	L	H	M	R	S	C	J
D	R	N	L	M	T	E	D	Y	R	D	K	C	B	Q
N	T	K	M	E	L	N	L	L	R	T	N	E	R	K
U	L	D	V	O	N	T	J	L	I	P	T	P	L	N
A	T	M	H	B	M	A	J	W	C	T	K	T	R	P
J	N	C	F	G	Z	Z	R	Y	J	K	M	I	T	T
L	R	P	S	U	L	U	V	L	O	V	H	O	T	T
B	L	M	L	N	L	N	J	M	K	L	R	N	X	L

1. ______________________ refers to chronic liver disease.
2. ______________________ means "inflammation of the gallbladder."
3. ______________________ means "varicose veins in the rectum."
4. ____________ occurs when one section of intestine telescopes into another section.
5. The term ____________ describes very dark, tarry stools due to presence of blood.
6. ______________________ is feeling the urge to vomit.
7. ______________ occurs when a length of bowel becomes twisted around itself.
8. ______________________ is a term describing the accumulation of fluid in the abdominal cavity.
9. ______________ refers to the yellow skin color associated with liver disease.
10. Esophageal ______________________ are varicose veins in the esophagus.

WORKSHEET 8F

Crossword Puzzle

Directions: Use the definitions to complete the crossword puzzles.

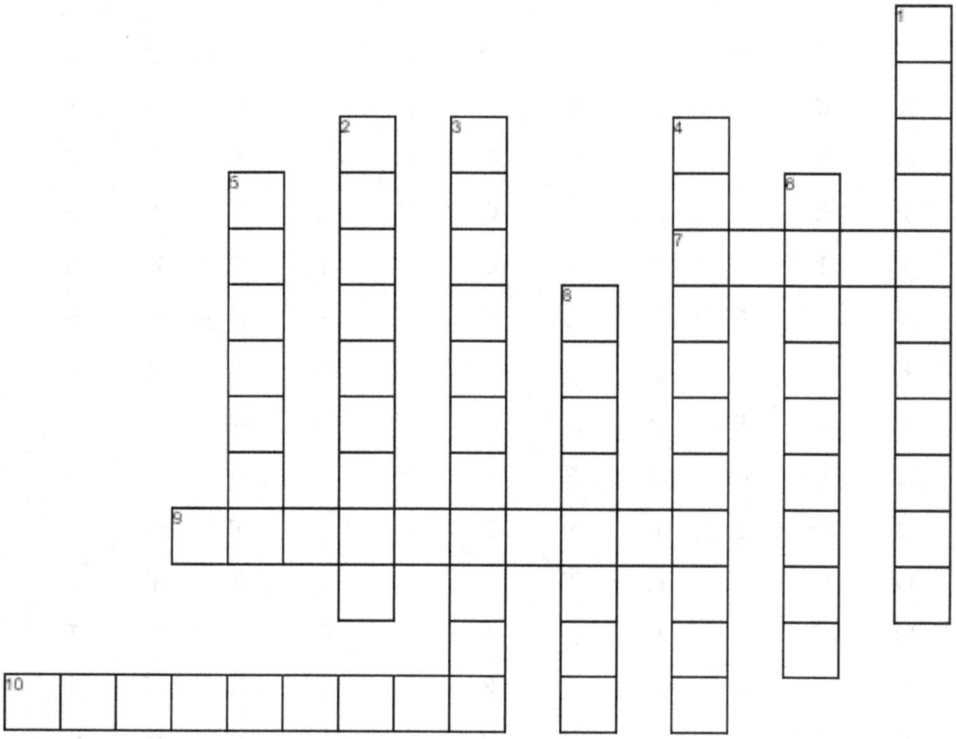

ACROSS

7 /o, the combining form for rectum and anus

9 Term meaning "pertaining to the pancreas"

10 Term meaning "inflammation of small intestine"

DOWN

1 Term meaning "vomiting blood"

2 /o, the combining form for common bile duct

3 Term meaning "excessive vomiting"

4 Term meaning "procedure to visually examine abdominal cavity"

5 Term meaning "without eating"

6 Term meaning "abnormal condition of having polyps"

8 Term meaning "liver tumor"

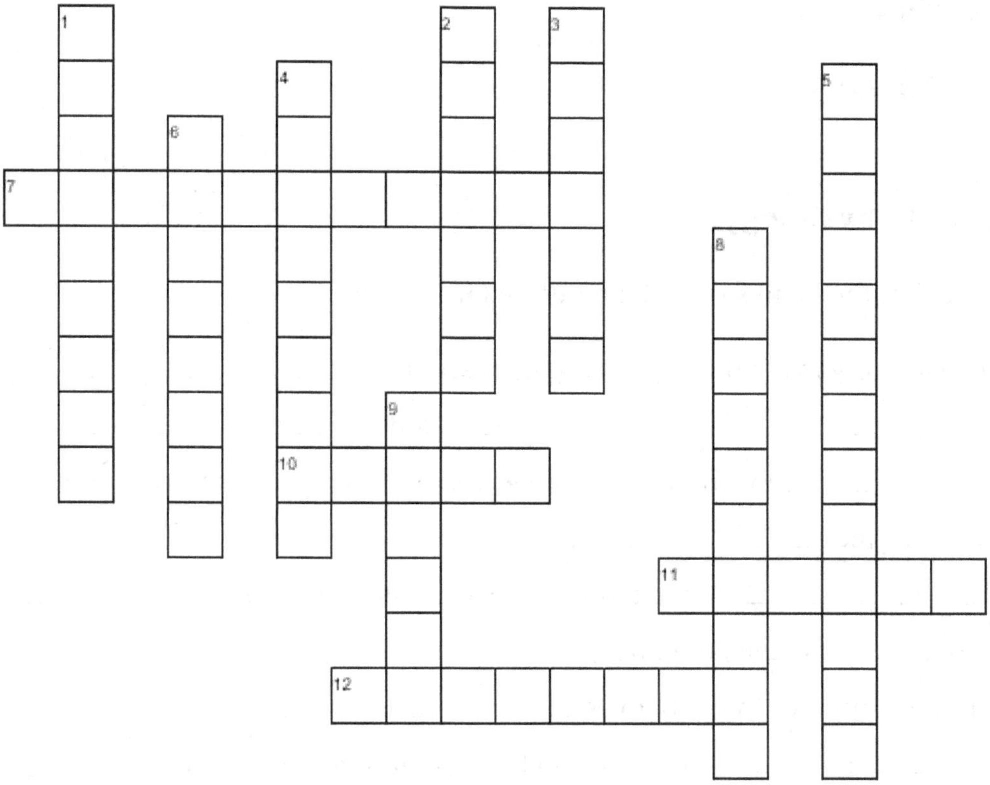

ACROSS

7 Varicose veins in the rectum

10 Occurs when food stops moving through digestive tract

11 ____________________ enema is also called a lower GI series

12 Yellow-colored skin from liver disease

DOWN

1 Symptoms include pain, diarrhea, and blood in stools

2 Accumulation of fluid in abdominal cavity

3 IBS is also called ____________________ colon

4 Chronic liver disease that can cause jaundice

5 Term meaning "gallbladder inflammation"

6 Length of bowel twisted around itself

8 A(n) ____________________ ulcer extends all the way through the stomach wall

9 Dark, tarry stools

WORKSHEET 8G

Chapter Review

Anatomy and Physiology

Directions: Fill in the blanks with the requested information.

1. The accessory organs of the digestive system are the ____________________, ____________________, ____________________, and ____________________.
2. ____________________ is the watery, slippery secretion in the oral cavity that contains the digestive enzyme, ____________________.
3. The ____________________ of a tooth is above the gum line and the ____________________ of the tooth is below the gum line.
4. The hardest substance in the body is ____________________.
5. The ____________________ prevents food from entering the trachea.
6. The stomach secretes ____________________.
7. ____________________ are rings of muscles that control entry into or exit from an organ.
8. The three sections of the small intestine are the ____________________, ____________________, and ____________________.
9. The appendix is attached to the ____________________ of the colon.
10. The liver secretes ____________________ to emulsify fats.

Word Building

Directions: Build a term for each of the following items.

1. inflammation of appendix ____________________
2. removal of gallbladder ____________________
3. create opening in colon ____________________
4. specialist in stomach and small intestine ____________________
5. instrument to view inside sigmoid colon ____________________
6. incision into abdomen ____________________
7. pertaining to straight teeth ____________________

8. surgical repair of palate ____________________

9. vomiting blood ____________________

10. slow digestion ____________________

Matching

Directions: Match the term with its definition.

_____ **1.** ascites	**a.** Tooth cavity
_____ **2.** cachexia	**b.** Gallstones
_____ **3.** crown	**c.** Yellow tint to the skin
_____ **4.** caries	**d.** Varicose veins in rectum
_____ **5.** emesis	**e.** Test for microscopic blood in stools
_____ **6.** hematochezia	**f.** Heartburn
_____ **7.** jaundice	**g.** Withdrawing fluid from abdominal cavity
_____ **8.** melena	**h.** Accumulation of fluid in peritoneal cavity
_____ **9.** polyp	**i.** Washing out the stomach
_____ **10.** pyrosis	**j.** Intestine twisted on itself
_____ **11.** aphthous ulcer	**k.** Dark, tarry stools
_____ **12.** herpes labialis	**l.** Diaphragmatocele
_____ **13.** hemorrhoids	**m.** X-ray to visualize bile ducts
_____ **14.** fistula	**n.** Bright red blood in the stools
_____ **15.** hiatal hernia	**o.** Treatment for morbid obesity
_____ **16.** intussusception	**p.** A diagnostic blood test
_____ **17.** volvulus	**q.** Loss of weight and generalized wasting
_____ **18.** cholelithiasis	**r.** Abnormal tube-like passageway
_____ **19.** ALT	**s.** Canker sore
_____ **20.** lavage	**t.** Small tumor on a stem or pedicle
_____ **21.** bariatric surgery	**u.** Artificial covering for tooth
_____ **22.** antiemetic	**v.** Treats nausea
_____ **23.** FOBT	**w.** Telescoping stretch of intestine
_____ **24.** paracentesis	**x.** Fever blister
_____ **25.** PTC	**y.** Vomiting

QUIZ 8A

New Word Parts Quiz

Directions: Define the combining form or suffix in the spaces provided.

1. bar/o ______
2. append/o ______
3. cholecyst/o ______
4. cec/o ______
5. dent/o ______
6. chol/e ______
7. hepat/o ______
8. lingu/o ______
9. gastr/o ______
10. proct/o ______
11. pharyng/o ______
12. cholangi/o ______
13. sialaden/o ______
14. or/o ______
15. odont/o ______
16. choledoch/o ______
17. gingiv/o ______
18. gloss/o ______
19. colon/o ______
20. enter/o ______
21. labi/o ______
22. –tripsy ______
23. -pepsia ______
24. –prandial ______
25. -phagia ______

QUIZ 8B

Labeling Diagram

Directions: Label the organs of the digestive system.

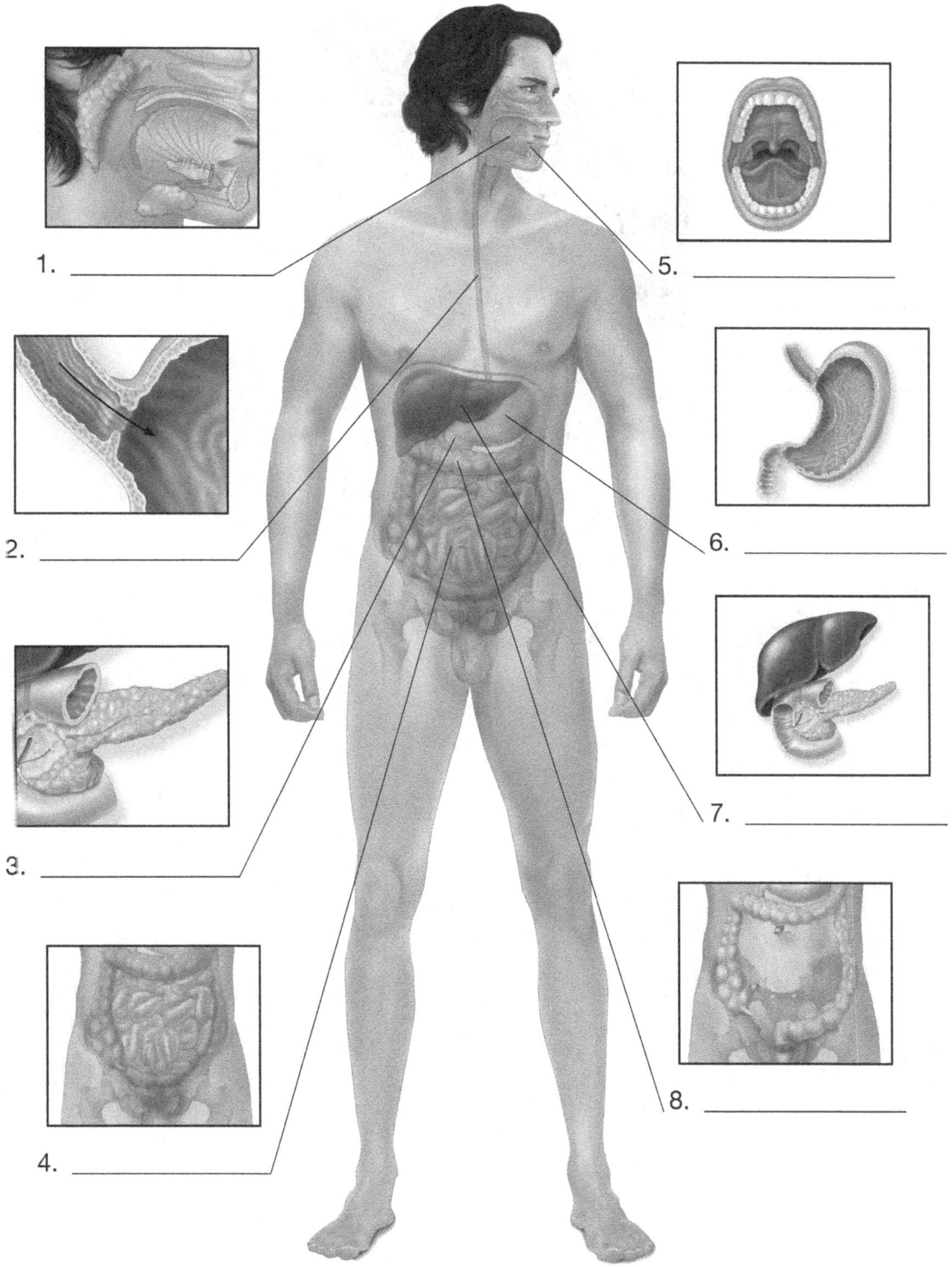

QUIZ 8C

Labeling Diagram

Directions: Label the organs of the digestive system.

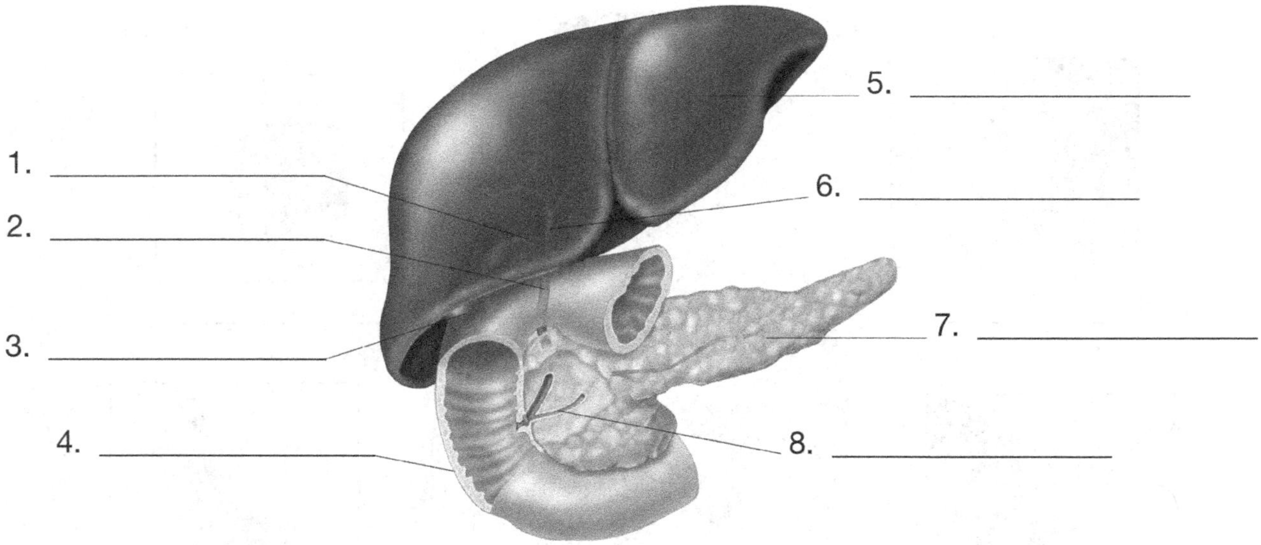

QUIZ 8D

Word Building Quiz

Directions: Build a single medical term for each phrase below.

1. pertaining to the anus ______
2. pertaining to the cheeks ______
3. pertaining to the gallbladder ______
4. pertaining to the colon ______
5. pertaining to teeth ______
6. pertaining to the duodenum ______
7. pertaining to the small intestine ______
8. pertaining to the esophagus ______
9. pertaining to the stomach ______
10. pertaining to the gums ______
11. pertaining to the liver ______
12. pertaining to the ileum ______
13. pertaining to the jejunum ______
14. pertaining to under the tongue ______
15. pertaining to the mouth ______
16. pertaining to the pancreas ______
17. pertaining to the throat ______
18. pertaining to the pylorus ______
19. pertaining to the rectum ______
20. abnormal appetite ______
21. excessive vomiting ______
22. slow digestion ______
23. unable to eat/swallow ______
24. after a meal ______
25. removal of the appendix ______

QUIZ 8E

Abbreviations Quiz

Directions: Write the medical term for which each abbreviation stands.

1. ac ______
2. Ba ______
3. BS ______
4. CBD ______
5. ERCP ______
6. FOBT ______
7. GB ______
8. GERD ______
9. GI ______
10. HCl ______
11. IBD ______
12. IVC ______
13. NG ______
14. NPO ______
15. n&v ______
16. O&P ______
17. pc ______
18. pp ______
19. TPN ______
20. PUD ______
21. UGI ______
22. PO ______
23. AST ______
24. BE ______
25. HAV ______

QUIZ 8F

Chapter Review

PART I: Multiple Choice

Directions: Circle the correct answer.

1. What is the medical term for the return of fluids and solids from the stomach into the mouth?
   a. dyspepsia
   b. regurgitation
   c. dysphagia
   d. aphagia
2. A protrusion of the stomach through the diaphragm and into the thoracic cavity is a(n)
   a. inguinal hernia.
   b. hiatal hernia.
   c. abdominal hernia.
   d. disk hernia.
3. The organ that produces bile is the
   a. gallbladder.
   b. pancreas.
   c. liver.
   d. small intestine.
4. The pathological condition characterized by twisting of the intestine on itself is called
   a. polyp.
   b. intussusception.
   c. volvulus.
   d. Crohn's disease.
5. The term for chronic disease of the liver with gradual destruction of its cells is
   a. dyspepsia.
   b. cirrhosis.
   c. peptic ulcer.
   d. volvulus.
6. The term for a series of X-rays taken of the stomach and duodenum after barium has been swallowed is
   a. lower GI.
   b. upper GI.
   c. anastomosis.
   d. retrograde cholangiography.
7. What is the medical term for tooth decay?
   a. ascites
   b. fistula
   c. gingivitis
   d. caries
8. Which surgical term listed below means to create a connection between two organs?
   a. gastrectomy
   b. anastomosis
   c. lithotripsy
   d. laparotomy

9. Which treatment listed below involves using a nasogastric tube to place a nutritional liquid into the stomach?

a. lavage
b. anastomosis
c. gavage
d. fistulectomy

10. Which of the following conditions is the presence of outpouches off the gut?

a. diverticulosis
b. polyposis
c. diaphragmatocele
d. ileus

PART II: Matching

Directions: Match the term with its definition.

____ **1.** chyme	**a.** Difficulty with defecation
____ **2.** cuspid	**b.** Treats gum conditions
____ **3.** constipation	**c.** An autoimmune condition
____ **4.** jaundice	**d.** An X-ray of the teeth
____ **5.** periodontics	**e.** Liquefied food leaving the stomach
____ **6.** cleft palate	**f.** To surgically pull teeth
____ **7.** Crohn's disease	**g.** A symptom of liver disease
____ **8.** bitewing	**h.** Treats peptic ulcers
____ **9.** extraction	**i.** A biting tooth
____ **10.** proton pump inhibitor	**j.** A congenital condition

PART III: Abbreviations

Directions: Write the full meaning of the following abbreviations.

1. PUD ______________________________

2. IBS ______________________________

3. NPO ______________________________

4. n&v ______________________________

5. EGD ______________________________

Chapter 9

Urinary System

Learning Objectives

Upon completion of this chapter, you will be able to:

- Identify and define the combining forms and suffixes introduced in this chapter.
- Correctly spell and pronounce medical terms and major anatomical structures relating to the urinary system.
- Locate and describe the major organs of the urinary system and their functions.
- Describe the nephron and the mechanisms of urine production.
- Identify the characteristics of urine and a urinalysis.
- Identify and define urinary system anatomical terms.
- Identify and define selected urinary system pathology terms.
- Identify and define selected urinary system diagnostic procedures.
- Identify and define selected urinary system therapeutic procedures.
- Identify and define selected medications relating to the urinary system.
- Define selected abbreviations associated with the urinary system.

WORKSHEET 9A

New Combining Form and Suffix

Directions: For each word part below, write its meaning. Then, locate a term from the chapter that uses the word part and its meaning.

Combining Forms	Meaning	Chapter Term	Meaning
1. azot/o			
2. bacteri/o			
3. cyst/o			
4. glomerul/o			
5. glycos/o			
6. home/o			
7. hydr/o			
8. keton/o			
9. meat/o			
10. nephr/o			
11. noct/I			
12. olig/o			
13. protein/o			
14. pyel/o			
15. ren/o			
16. ureter/o			
17. urethr/o			
18. urin/o			
19. ur/o			

Suffixes

20. –lith			
21. –lysis			
22. –ptosis			
23. –uria			

WORKSHEET 9B

Medical Term Analysis

Directions: Below are terms built from word parts used in this chapter that are not analyzed in the Word Building Table. Many are built from word parts you have learned in previous chapters. Analyze each term presented below by listing and defining each of the word parts used to build each term.

Medical Term	**Word Part Analysis**
1. necrosis	________________
2. antibiotic	________________
3. azotemia	________________
4. cystocele	________________
5. cystography	________________
6. cystoscopy	________________
7. urography	________________
8. Glomerular	________________
9. glomerulonephritis	________________
10. hydronephrosis	________________
11. intravenous	________________
12. meatotomy	________________
13. nephrolithotomy	________________
14. nephrology	________________
15. nephrotic	________________
16. neurogenic	________________
17. cystoplasty	________________
18. polycystic	________________
19. pyelonephritis	________________
20. carcinoma	________________
21. retroperitoneal	________________
22. uremia	________________
23. urinalysis	________________
24. urography	________________
25. urology	________________
26. cystourethrography	________________

WORKSHEET 9C

Unscramble

Directions: Unscramble each medical term below. A definition for the term is given below each scrambled term.

1. n i r u y i s a l s ____________________

   Physical, chemical, and microscopic examination of urine

2. l e y d o i s h m a s i ____________________

   Using artificial kidney machine to filter waste from blood

3. t a h c t e i r e a t i z n o ____________________

   Inserting flexible tube into bladder

4. r u i a p y ____________________

   Pus in the urine

5. o n e h p r n ____________________

   Functional working unit of kidney

6. s t a o c l p t y s y ____________________

   Surgical repair of bladder

7. s e h i t n a y c ____________________

   Decrease in force of urine stream

8. e n p i r o p h t o s s ____________________

   Also known as floating kidney

9. s c l u c l u a ____________________

   A stone

10. a i t l r t o n i f ____________________

    First stage of urine production

WORKSHEET 9D

Sound It Out

Directions: The following are some of the important terms from this chapter written as their phonetic spellings. Sound out each term and write it in the blank.

1. yoo-ree-ter-oh-sten-OH-sis ______
2. yoo-RAL-oh-jee ______
3. yoo-rin-OH-meter ______
4. neh-FROH-ma ______
5. dis-YOO-ree-ah ______
6. en-yoo-REE-sis ______
7. hee-mah-TOO-ree-ah ______
8. hee-moh-dye-AL-ih-sis ______
9. pye-eh-loh-neh-FRYE-tis ______
10. SIS-toh-lith ______
11. LITH-oh-trip-see ______
12. mee-AY-tus ______
13. nef-roh-skleh-ROH-sis ______
14. nok-TOO-ree-ah ______
15. pol-ee-YOO-ree-ah ______
16. yoo-REE-ter ______
17. pye-YOO-ree-ah ______
18. yoo-REE-thral ______
19. KAL-kew-lus ______
20. yoo-REE-mee-ah ______
21. sis-TEK-toh-me ______
22. yoo-REE-throh-scope ______
23. yoo-rih-NAL-ih-sis ______
24. nef-roh-MEG-ah-lee ______
25. NEF-roh-pek-see ______

WORKSHEET 9E

Word Search Puzzle

Directions: Find and circle the answer for each fill-in-the-blank question in the word search puzzle.

I	N	C	O	N	T	I	N	E	N	C	E	Z
K	C	Y	H	T	A	P	O	R	H	P	E	N
C	Y	S	N	N	N	M	T	V	H	R	X	S
R	S	P	S	H	P	L	V	Z	L	L	I	H
E	T	I	U	N	E	N	T	J	M	S	M	U
A	O	R	L	D	Y	S	X	K	Y	Q	R	V
T	P	T	U	W	H	T	I	L	C	G	C	G
I	E	O	C	G	K	V	A	T	E	D	M	B
N	X	H	L	X	D	N	G	N	A	P	X	X
I	Y	T	A	G	I	D	C	R	Y	N	B	X
N	D	I	C	R	T	Y	W	N	T	X	C	Q
E	Q	L	U	W	L	D	M	Q	C	T	T	Y
F	R	E	Q	U	E	N	C	Y	G	R	Q	H

1. Another term for a stone is ____________________.
2. A(n) ____________________ is a physical and chemical analysis of urine.
3. Feeling the urge to urinate more often than normal is called ____________________.
4. Difficulty initiating the flow of urine is called ____________________.
5. ____________________ is the surgical fixation of the bladder.
6. The involuntary release of urine is called ____________________.
7. Diabetic ____________________ is damage to glomerular capillaries caused by diabetes.
8. ____________________ clearance is a test of kidney function.
9. ____________________ is the surgical crushing of a stone.
10. ____________________ is feeling the need to urinate immediately.

WORKSHEET 9F

Crossword Puzzle

Directions: Use the definitions to complete the crossword puzzles.

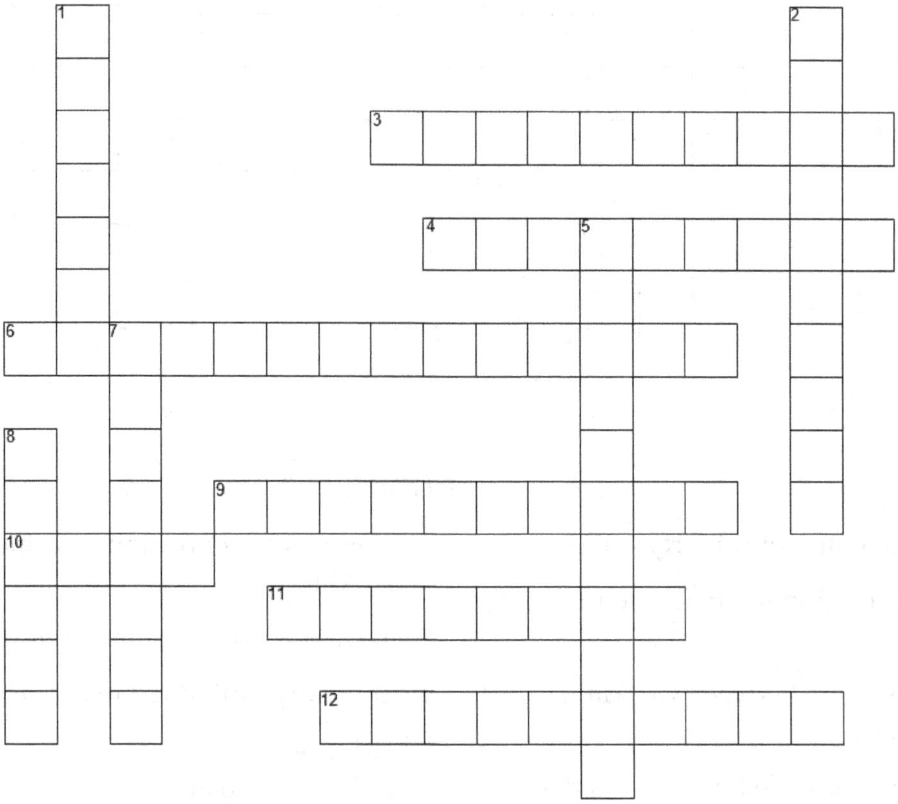

ACROSS

3 Medication used to treat bacterial infections

4 Retrograde ____________________ is an X-ray of the urinary tract using dye

6 Inflammation of renal pelvis and kidney

9 kidneys have multiple cysts

10 A BUN tests for the level of ____________________ in the blood

11 Term meaning "scanty amount of urine"

12 Instrument used to visually examine inside the bladder

DOWN

1 Need to urinate immediately

2 Laboratory test to examine urine

5 Surgical procedure to crush a stone

7 Another term for urinary incontinence

8 Term meaning "pus in the urine"

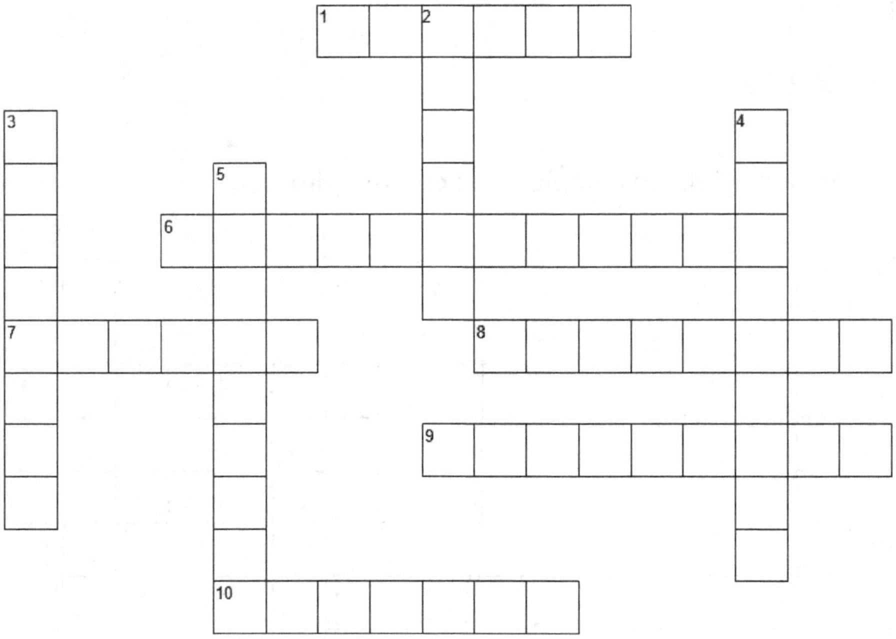

ACROSS

1 External opening of the urethra

6 Using artificial kidney machine to filter waste

7 Transports urine between the kidney and the bladder

8 Flexible tube inserted into the bladder

9 Urge to urinate more often than normal

10 Functional working unit of kidney

DOWN

2 Complete suppression of urine formed by kidneys

3 Term for a stone formed within an organ

4 Difficulty initiating flow of urine

5 Urinary __________________, inability to fully empty bladder

WORKSHEET 9G

Chapter Review

Anatomy and Physiology

Directions: Fill in the blanks with the requested information.

1. The organs of the urinary system are the ____________________, ____________________, ____________________, and ____________________.
2. The functional unit of the kidneys is the ____________________.
3. The main function of the urinary system is to ____________________.
4. The outer region of the kidney is the ____________________ and the inner region is the
5. The renal corpuscle consists of the ____________________ and ____________________ .
6. The kidneys are responsible for ____________________ or balance in the body.
7. The three stages of urine production are ____________________, ____________________, and ____________________.
8. ____________________ indicates the amount of dissolved substances in the urine.
9. Urine is normally ____________________ colored and 95 percent ____________________.
10. Urine is carried from the kidneys to the bladder in the ____________________ and from the bladder to the outside of the body in the ____________________.

Word Building

Directions: Build a term for each of the following items.

1. excision of the bladder ____
2. bladder pain ____
3. surgical crushing of a stone ____
4. kidney softening ____
5. kidney tumor ____
6. kidney disease ____
7. ureter stone ____
8. narrowing of the urethra ____

9. condition of sugar in the urine ____________________

10. condition of pus in the urine ____________________

Matching

Directions: Match the term with its definition.

____ **1.** calculus	**a.** Protrusion of bladder into vaginal wall
____ **2.** urgency	**b.** Urinalysis
____ **3.** enuresis	**c.** Decrease in the force of the urine stream
____ **4.** micturition	**d.** A flat abdomen X-ray
____ **5.** hesitancy	**e.** Commonly seen in children
____ **6.** hydronephrosis	**f.** Medication to increase urine volume
____ **7.** nephroptosis	**g.** Involuntary discharge of urine
____ **8.** Cystocele	**h.** Artificial filtering of waste from blood
____ **9.** renal failure	**i.** May be caused by spinal cord injury
____ **10.** Wilm's tumor	**j.** Treatment for kidney stones
____ **11.** neurogenic bladder	**k.** X-ray of renal pelvis
____ **12.** hematuria	**l.** Stone
____ **13.** BUN	**m.** Implantation of a donor kidney
____ **14.** U/A	**n.** Accumulation of urine in the renal pelvis
____ **15.** IVP	**o.** Test that grows bacteria in a culture medium
____ **16.** urine C&S	**p.** Collects uncontaminated urine for testing
____ **17.** kidneys, ureter, bladder	**q.** Feeling the need to urinate immediately
____ **18.** cystoscopy	**r.** Blood in the urine
____ **19.** catheterization	**s.** Medication to treat bacterial infection
____ **20.** hemodialysis	**t.** Floating kidney
____ **21.** ESWL	**u.** Insertion of a flexible tube into the bladder
____ **22.** renal transplant	**v.** Another term for urination
____ **23.** clean catch specimen	**w.** Blood test for kidney function
____ **24.** antibiotic	**x.** Visual exam of the bladder
____ **25.** diuretic	**y.** Inability of the kidneys to filter waste

QUIZ 9A

New Word Parts Quiz

Directions: Define the combining form or suffix in the spaces provided.

1. azot/o ____________________
2. bacteri/o ____________________
3. cyst/o ____________________
4. glomerul/o ____________________
5. glycos/o ____________________
6. keton/o ____________________
7. lith/o ____________________
8. meat/o ____________________
9. nephr/o ____________________
10. noct/i ____________________
11. olig/o ____________________
12. pyel/o ____________________
13. ren/o ____________________
14. ur/o ____________________
15. ureter/o ____________________
16. urethr/o ____________________
17. urin/o ____________________
18. -lith ____________________
19. -ptosis ____________________
20. -uria ____________________

QUIZ 9B

Labeling Diagram

Directions: Label the structures of the urinary system.

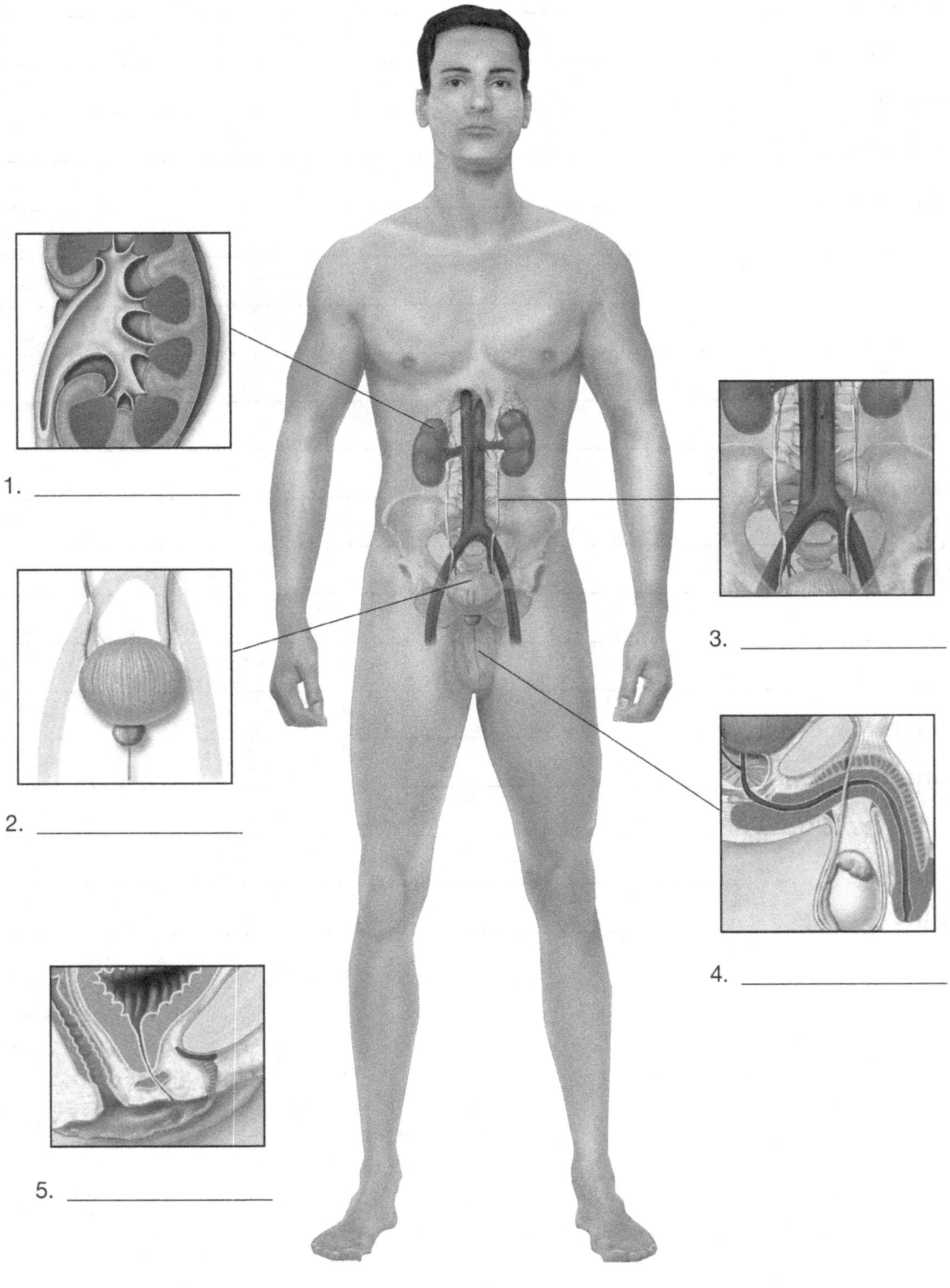

QUIZ 9C

Labeling Diagram

Directions: Label the internal structures of the kidney.

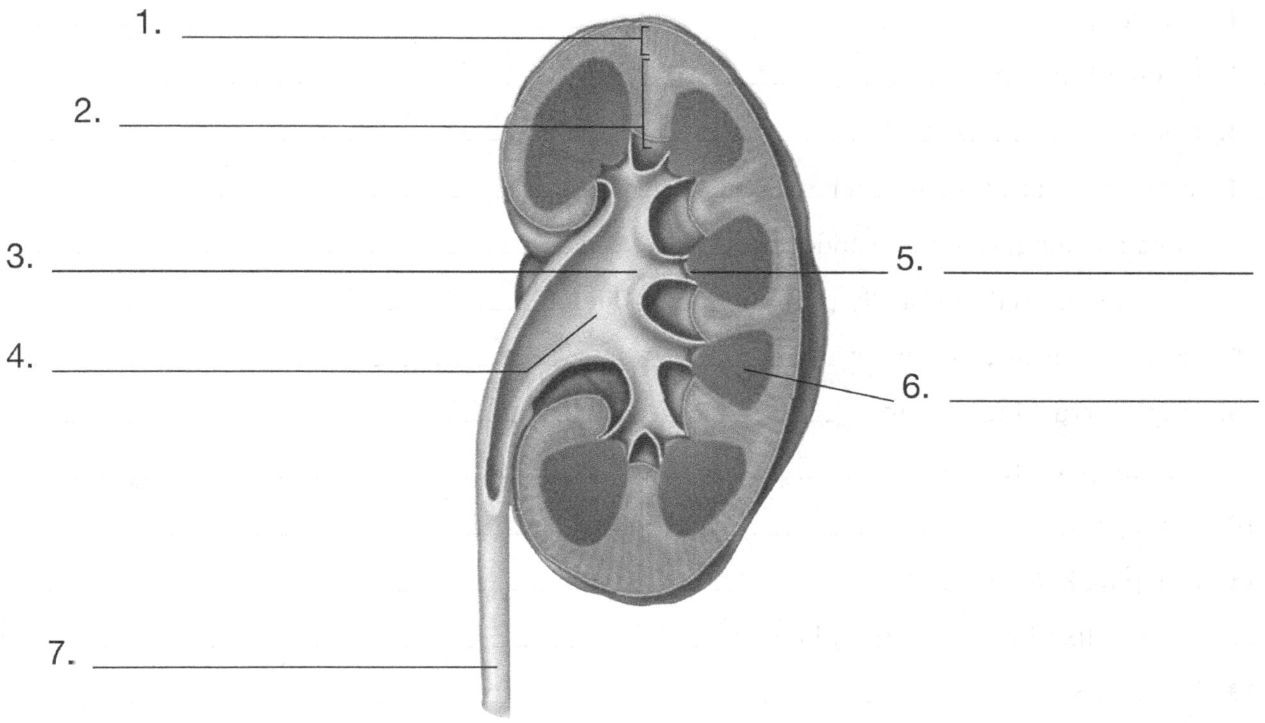

QUIZ 9D

Word Building Quiz

Directions: Build a single medical term for each phrase below.

1. bladder pain ____________________
2. bladder inflammation ____________________
3. bladder stone ____________________
4. surgical repair of the bladder ____________________
5. rapid bleeding from the bladder ____________________
6. instrument used to visually examine the bladder ____________________
7. condition of sugar in the urine ____________________
8. surgical crushing of a stone ____________________
9. softening of the kidney ____________________
10. kidney tumor ____________________
11. drooping kidney ____________________
12. surgical fixation of (floating) kidney ____________________
13. kidney disease ____________________
14. hardening of the kidney ____________________
15. condition of (frequent) nighttime urination ____________________
16. X-ray record of the renal pelvis ____________________
17. surgical repair of the renal pelvis ____________________
18. condition of pus in the urine ____________________
19. narrowing of a ureter ____________________
20. pertaining to the kidney ____________________
21. instrument to visually examine the urethra ____________________
22. condition of no urine (produced by kidney) ____________________
23. condition of difficult or painful urination ____________________
24. condition of blood in the urine ____________________
25. condition of (too) much urine ____________________

QUIZ 9E

Abbreviations Quiz

Directions: Write the medical term for which each abbreviation stands.

1. AGN ______
2. ARF ______
3. ATN ______
4. BNO ______
5. BUN ______
6. cath ______
7. Cl ______
8. CRF ______
9. C&S ______
10. cysto ______
11. ESWL ______
12. EU ______
13. HD ______
14. H2O ______
15. I&O ______
16. IVP ______
17. K+ ______
18. KUB ______
19. Na+ ______
20. RP ______
21. SG, sp. gr. ______
22. U/A, UA ______
23. UC ______
24. UTI ______
25. VCUG ______

QUIZ 9F

Chapter Review

PART I: Multiple Choice

Directions: Circle the correct answer.

1. Excision of a kidney is called
   - **a.** nephrectomy.
   - **b.** nephropexy.
   - **c.** nephrotomy.
   - **d.** pyeloplasty.
2. A distention of the renal pelvis due to urine collecting in the kidney, often the result of obstruction, is
   - **a.** nephrolithiasis.
   - **b.** hydronephrosis.
   - **c.** cystocele.
   - **d.** pyelonephritis.
3. In nephromegaly, there is
   - **a.** an enlargement in the kidney.
   - **b.** a stone present in the kidney.
   - **c.** an inflammation of the kidney.
   - **d.** a prolapse of the kidney.
4. The abbreviation UTI stands for
   - **a.** urethral toxic infection.
   - **b.** ureter total inflammation.
   - **c.** urinary tract incontinence.
   - **d.** urinary tract infection.
5. The medical term for abnormal kidney condition is
   - **a.** nephroptosis.
   - **b.** nephrosis.
   - **c.** nephromalacia.
   - **d.** nephritis.
6. The act of voiding urine is called
   - **a.** nocturia.
   - **b.** micturition.
   - **c.** oliguria.
   - **d.** urodynia.
7. What is inflammation of the bladder called?
   - **a.** nephritis
   - **b.** urinary tract infection
   - **c.** cystitis
   - **d.** pyelitis

8. What is the use of an artificial kidney machine to filter the blood of a person to remove waste products called?

a. catheterization
b. hemodialysis
c. azotemia
d. BUN

9. What is the medical term for ureteral narrowing?

a. ureterostenosis
b. ureterolysis
c. ureterosclerosis
d. urethrostenosis

10. What is the functional unit of the kidney?

a. glomerulus
b. renal tubule
c. nephron
d. renal corpuscle

PART II: Matching

Directions: Match the term with its definition.

_____	**1.** polyuria	**a.** Scanty amount of urine
_____	**2.** dysuria	**b.** Condition of blood in urine
_____	**3.** pyuria	**c.** Condition of too much urine
_____	**4.** oliguria	**d.** Condition of ketones in urine
_____	**5.** nocturia	**e.** Frequent nighttime urination
_____	**6.** enuresis	**f.** Difficult urination
_____	**7.** hematuria	**g.** Complete lack of urine secretion
_____	**8.** ketonuria	**h.** Condition of pus in urine
_____	**9.** anuria	**i.** Bed-wetting at night

PART III: Abbreviations

Directions: Write the full meaning of the following abbreviations.

1. BUN ____

2. GU ____

3. IVP ____

4. KUB ____

5. CRF ____

Chapter 10

Reproductive System

Learning Objectives

Upon completion of this chapter, you will be able to:

- Identify and define the combining forms, suffixes, and prefixes introduced in this chapter.
- Correctly spell and pronounce medical terms and major anatomical structures relating to the reproductive systems.
- Locate and describe the major organs of the reproductive systems and their functions.
- Use medical terms to describe circumstances relating to pregnancy.
- Identify and define reproductive system anatomical terms.
- Identify and define selected reproductive system pathology terms.
- Identify the symptoms and origin of sexually transmitted diseases.
- Identify and define selected reproductive system diagnostic procedures.
- Identify and define selected reproductive system therapeutic procedures.
- Identify and define selected medications relating to the reproductive systems.
- Define selected abbreviations associated with the reproductive systems.

WORKSHEET 10A

New Combining Form, Suffix, and Prefix

Directions: For each word part below, write its meaning. Then, locate a term from the chapter that uses the word part and its meaning.

Combining Forms	Meaning	Chapter Term	Meaning
1. amni/o	______	______	______
2. cervic/o	______	______	______
3. chori/o	______	______	______
4. colp/o	______	______	______
5. culd/o	______	______	______
6. dilat/o	______	______	______
7. embry/o	______	______	______
8. episi/o	______	______	______
9. estr/o	______	______	______
10. fet/o	______	______	______
11. gynec/o	______	______	______
12. hymen/o	______	______	______
13. hyster/o	______	______	______
14. lact/o	______	______	______
15. mamm/o	______	______	______
16. mast/o	______	______	______
17. men/o	______	______	______
18. metr/o	______	______	______
19. nat/o	______	______	______
20. o/o	______	______	______
21. oophor/o	______	______	______
22. ov/o, ov/i	______	______	______
23. ovari/o	______	______	______
24. pareun/o	______	______	______

25. perine/o ______ ______ ______
26. radic/o ______ ______ ______
27. salping/o ______ ______ ______
28. uter/o ______ ______ ______
29. vagin/o ______ ______ ______
30. vulv/o ______ ______ ______
31. andr/o ______ ______ ______
32. balan/o ______ ______ ______
33. crypt/o ______ ______ ______
34. epididym/o ______ ______ ______
35. orch/o ______ ______ ______
36. orchi/o ______ ______ ______
37. orchid/o ______ ______ ______
38. pen/o ______ ______ ______
39. prostat/o ______ ______ ______
40. spermat/o ______ ______ ______
41. testicul/o ______ ______ ______
42. vas/o ______ ______ ______
43. vesicul/o ______ ______ ______

Suffixes

44. –arche ______ ______ ______
45. –cyesis ______ ______ ______
46. –genesis ______ ______ ______
47. –gravida ______ ______ ______
48. –para ______ ______ ______
49. –partum ______ ______ ______
50. –salpinx ______ ______ ______
51. –tocia ______ ______ ______
52. –cide ______ ______ ______

53. –plasia ______________ ______________ ______________

54. –spermia ______________ ______________ ______________

Prefixes

55. ante- ______________ ______________ ______________

56. contra- ______________ ______________ ______________

57. primi- ______________ ______________ ______________

WORKSHEET 10B

Medical Term Analysis

Directions: Below are terms built from word parts used in this and previous chapters. Analyze each term presented below, and list and define the word parts used to build each term.

Medical Term **Word Part Analysis**

1. menarche ______
2. gynecology ______
3. intrauterine ______
4. neonatology ______
5. carcinoma ______
6. endometrial ______
7. menometrorrhagia ______
8. cystocele ______
9. endometriosis ______
10. hemolytic ______
11. hysterosalpingography ______
12. mammography ______
13. culdoscopy ______
14. laparoscopy ______
15. amniocentesis ______
16. biopsy ______
17. episiotomy ______
18. hysterectomy ______
19. oophorectomy ______
20. spermatogenesis ______
21. cryptorchidism ______
22. varicocele ______
23. vasovasostomy ______
24. vasectomy ______
25. transurethral ______

WORKSHEET 10C

Unscramble

Directions: Unscramble each medical term below. A definition for the term is given below each scrambled term.

1. o c i n n a i t o z ______________________

   Removal of core of cervical tissue for biopsy

2. t i e r l a f i z t n i o ______________________

   Joining of ova and sperm

3. r h c o o n i ______________________

   Outer sac protecting fetus

4. l e s o t c c y e ______________________

   Protrusion of bladder into vagina

5. g a s l a t i a m ______________________

   Breast pain

6. d u m o e r t i m e n ______________________

   Inner layer of the uterus

7. a y l m a h d i c ______________________

   Bacterial sexually transmitted disease

8. c a i r o v e c l e ______________________

   Varicose veins in scrotum

9. l a a h b o r n e a r ______________________

   Discharge from glans penis

10. c a e m v t o s y ______________________

    Surgical removal of vas deferens

WORKSHEET 10D

Sound It Out

Directions: The following are some of the important terms from this chapter written as their phonetic spellings. Sound out each term and write it in the blank.

1. am-nee-oh-sen-TEE-sis ______________________
2. kol-POS-koh-pee ______________________
3. SIS-toh-seel ______________________
4. dis-men-oh-REE-ah ______________________
5. en-doh-mee-tree-OH-sis ______________________
6. eh-peez-ee-OT-oh-mee ______________________
7. gigh-neh-KALL-oh-jee ______________________
8. hiss-ter-EK-toh-me ______________________
9. lap-ah-ROT-oh-mee ______________________
10. MAM-oh-gram ______________________
11. mas-TEK-toh-mee ______________________
12. mull-TIP-ah-rah ______________________
13. null-ih-GRAV-ih-dah ______________________
14. oh-of-or-EK-toh-mee ______________________
15. post-PAR-tum ______________________
16. bah-lah-noh-REE-ah ______________________
17. ah-SPER-mee-ah ______________________
18. ep-ih-did-ih-MY-tis ______________________
19. gon-oh-REE-ah ______________________
20. fye-MOH-sis ______________________
21. or-kih-DEK-toh-mee ______________________
22. sper-mah-TALL-ih-sis ______________________
23. pross-tah-TYE-tis ______________________
24. tess-TIK-yoo-lar ______________________
25. vah-SEK-toh-mee ______________________

WORKSHEET 10E

Word Search Puzzle

Directions: Find and circle the answer for each fill-in-the-blank question in the word search puzzle.

L	H	E	N	D	O	M	E	T	R	I	O	S	I	S
M	R	R	N	K	N	J	J	H	Y	N	T	F	N	N
F	Q	A	Q	B	N	Q	Y	L	H	R	F	A	G	C
Z	H	N	L	Q	M	D	T	T	B	K	I	K	D	I
W	X	L	T	U	R	Z	R	R	D	C	H	H	Q	R
Z	L	W	G	O	C	I	G	R	I	L	M	M	P	C
V	Z	R	C	Z	B	I	P	R	B	K	M	B	Z	U
K	M	E	E	L	C	N	T	R	Q	M	C	D	J	M
Z	L	T	L	C	I	E	T	S	P	M	I	J	R	C
E	G	I	N	M	T	B	G	C	E	T	P	F	P	I
Z	T	K	L	S	O	O	P	M	Y	T	O	X	B	S
S	B	P	B	G	I	C	C	W	L	F	T	G	C	I
B	K	O	L	M	N	J	N	E	D	V	C	M	X	O
F	S	I	S	O	M	I	H	P	L	N	E	L	F	N
W	J	V	B	K	A	M	B	H	T	E	F	V	T	M

1. A(n) ______________________ pregnancy occurs outside the uterus.
2. A(n) ______________________ is the death of a viable-aged fetus.
3. ______________________ occurs when endometrial tissue appears throughout the pelvic or abdominal cavity.
4. ______________________ are physicians who specialize in pregnancy and childbirth.
5. The fetus floats in ______________________ fluid.
6. A protrusion of the rectum into the vagina is called a(n) ______________________.
7. ______________________ is the removal of the prepuce.
8. ______________________ is the accumulation of fluid within the scrotum.
9. A narrowing of the prepuce of the glans penis is called ______________________.
10. ______________________ cancer is commonly seen in young men or boys.

WORKSHEET 10F

Crossword Puzzle

Directions: Use the definitions to complete the crossword puzzles.

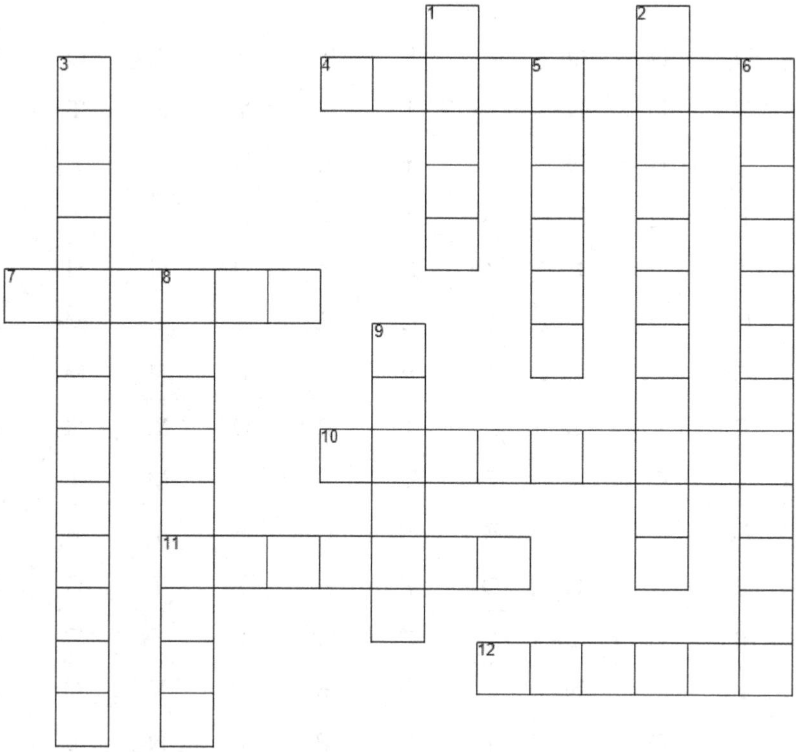

ACROSS

4 Release of ovum from ovary

7 Early stage of human development, ends at second month

10 Term meaning "first birth"

11 Outer sac around the fetus

12 Organ also called birth canal

DOWN

1 Term referring to the external genitalia of the female

2 Another term for spontaneous abortion

3 Endometrial tissue appears throughout pelvic cavity

5 Inner sac around the fetus

6 Term meaning "no pregnancies"

8 Herniation of rectum into vagina

9 Narrow region of uterus, opens into vagina

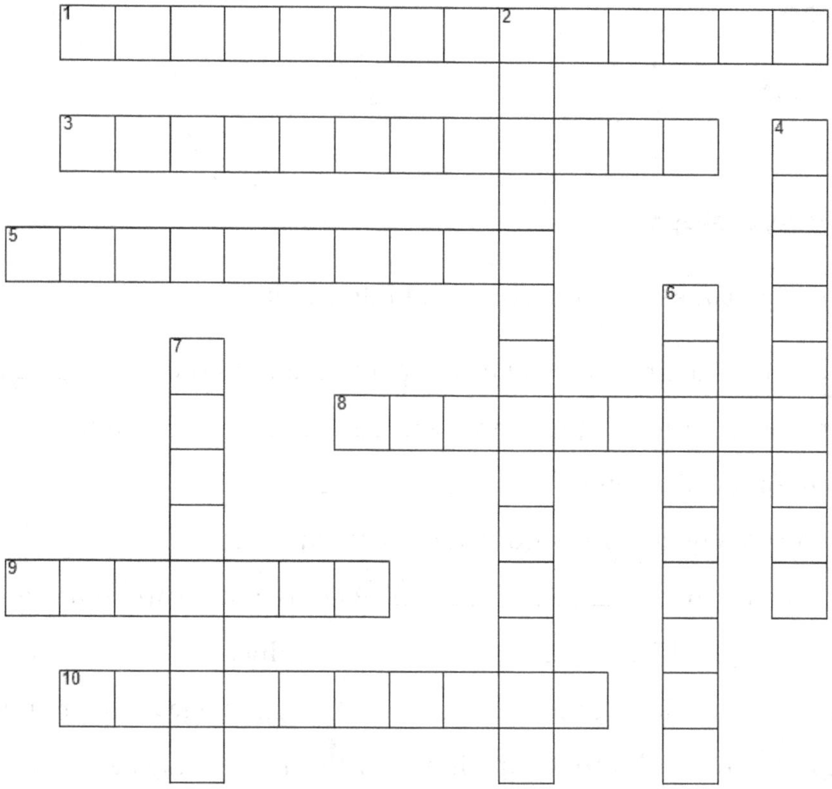

ACROSS

1 Another term for undescended testicle

3 Surgical removal of prepuce

5 Enlarged veins in spermatic cord

8 Accumulation of fluid within scrotum

9 Testes are suspended outside the body in the ___________________

10 Organ that stores sperm made by the testes

DOWN

2 Term meaning "ruptured uterus"

4 Another term for erectile dysfunction

6 Inability to produce children

7 Narrowing of prepuce over glans penis

WORKSHEET 10G

Chapter Review

Anatomy and Physiology

Directions: Fill in the blanks with the requested information.

1. The female external genitalia are collectively referred to as the ____________________.
2. The sex hormones secreted by the ovaries are __________________ and __________________.
3. Another term for fertilization is ____________________.
4. The uterus is normally bent forward, which is called ____________________.
5. Milk is produced by the ____________________ glands and is carried to the ____________________ by the ____________________ ducts.
6. The infant is delivered during the ____________________ stage of labor and delivery.
7. Appearance of the baby's buttocks first in the birth canal is called a ____________________ presentation.
8. ____________________ is the process of producing sperm.
9. ____________________ is the release of semen into the female vagina.
10. The ____________________ is covered by the ____________________ or foreskin.

Word Building

Directions: Build a term for each of the following items.

1. instrument to view inside abdomen ____
2. ruptured uterus ____
3. pus in uterine tube ____
4. before birth ____
5. false pregnancy ____
6. flow from uterus ____
7. surgical repair of glans penis ____
8. surgical fixation of testes ____

9. removal of prostate ____________________

10. condition of scanty sperm ____________________

Matching

Directions: Match the term with its definition.

_____ **1.** infertility	**a.** May be caused by human papillomavirus
_____ **2.** condom	**b.** Obtains a core of cervical tissue
_____ **3.** colostrum	**c.** Convulsions and coma during pregnancy
_____ **4.** oxytocin	**d.** Narrowing of prepuce
_____ **5.** menarche	**e.** Hormone that improves uterine contractions
_____ **6.** cervical cancer	**f.** Reverses a vasectomy
_____ **7.** prolapsed	**g.** Spontaneous abortion
_____ **8.** PID	**h.** First menstrual period
_____ **9.** eclampsia	**i.** Test for cervical cancer
_____ **10.** HDN	**j.** Venereal ulcer
_____ **11.** abruptio placentae	**k.** First milk secreted from breast
_____ **12.** stillbirth	**l.** pregnancy in the uterine tube
_____ **13.** Pap smear	**m.** Undescended testicle
_____ **14.** miscarriage	**n.** Placenta tears away from uterine wall
_____ **15.** amniocentesis	**o.** Inability to produce children
_____ **16.** conization	**p.** Impotence
_____ **17.** tubal ligation	**q.** Also called erythroblastosis fetalis
_____ **18.** salpingocyesis	**r.** Fallen uterus
_____ **19.** cryptorchidism	**s.** Persistent erection
_____ **20.** erectile dysfunction	**t.** Test for genetic abnormalities
_____ **21.** phimosis	**u.** Example of barrier contraception
_____ **22.** priapism	**v.** Blood test for prostate cancer
_____ **23.** chancroid	**w.** Death of a viable-aged fetus
_____ **24.** PSA	**x.** Usually bacterial infection of pelvic cavity
_____ **25.** vasovasostomy	**y.** Sterilization procedure

QUIZ 10A

New Word Parts Quiz

Directions: Define the combining form or suffix in the spaces provided.

1. colp/o ______
2. episi/o ______
3. gynec/o ______
4. hyster/o ______
5. lact/o ______
6. amni/o ______
7. metr/o ______
8. mamm/o ______
9. salping/o ______
10. perine/o ______
11. nat/o ______
12. oophor/o ______
13. vas/o ______
14. andr/o ______
15. crypt/o ______
16. balan/o ______
17. orch/o ______
18. vesicul/o ______
19. varic/o ______
20. testicul/o ______
21. –arche ______
22. –salpinx ______
23. –tocia ______
24. –gravida ______
25. –spermia ______

QUIZ 10B

Labeling Diagram

Directions: Label the components of the female reproductive system.

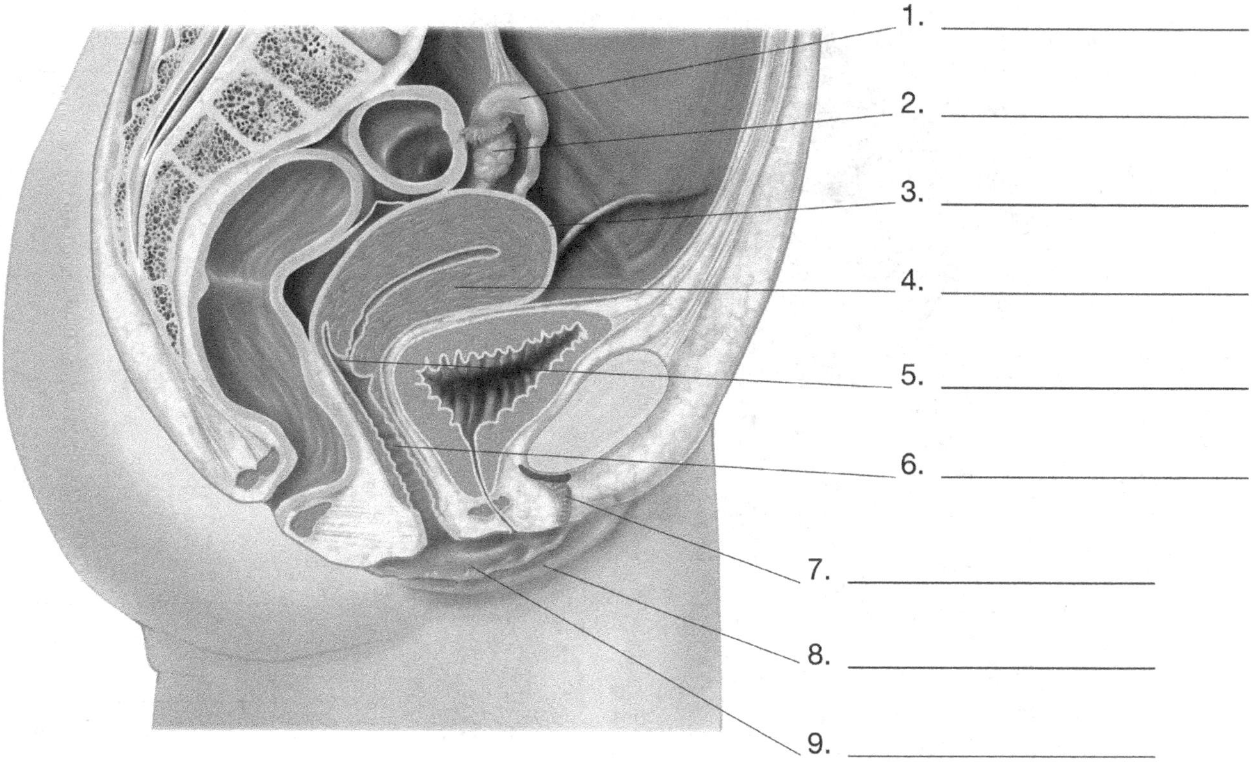

QUIZ 10C

Labeling Diagram

Directions: Label the organs of the male reproductive system.

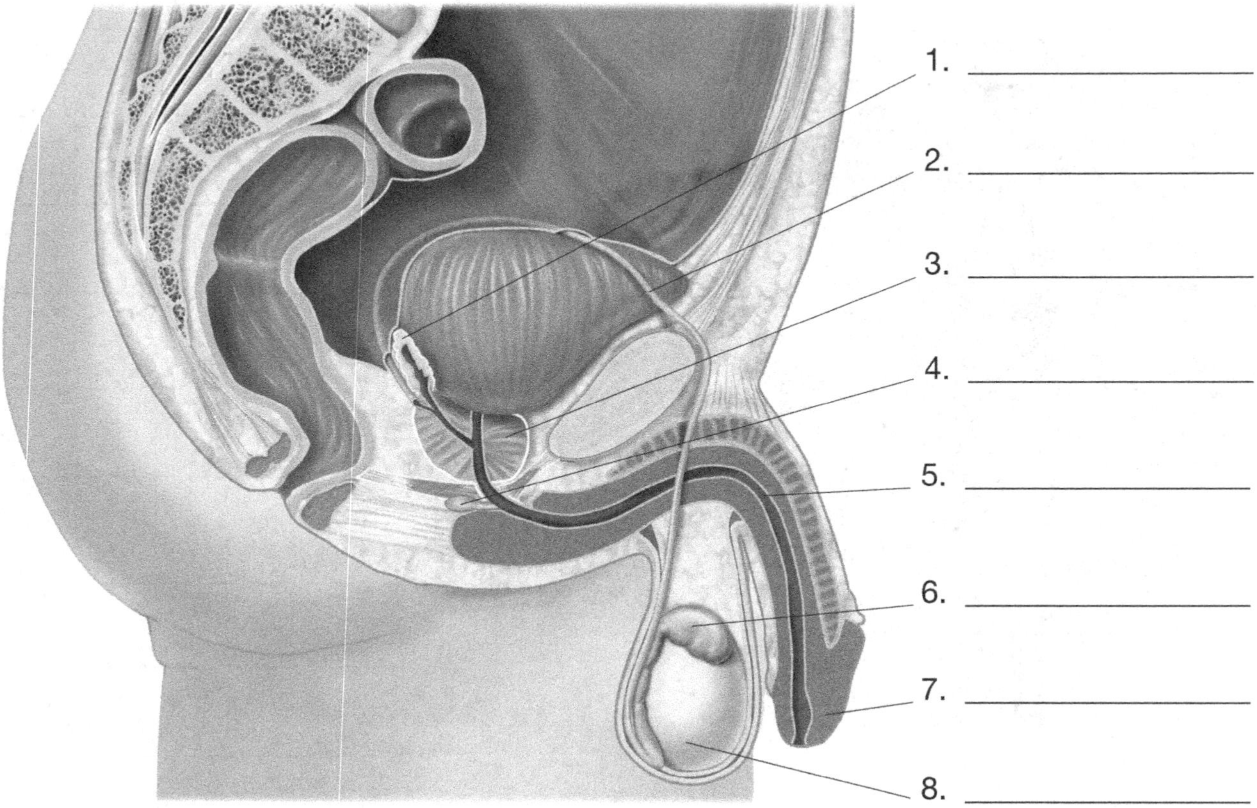

QUIZ 10D

Word Building Quiz

Directions: Build a single medical term for each phrase below.

1. pertaining to amnion ______
2. removal of cervix ______
3. instrument to view inside vagina ______
4. pertaining to embryo ______
5. suture of vulva ______
6. surgical fixation of uterus ______
7. breast pain ______
8. record of breast ______
9. no menstrual flow ______
10. milk discharge ______
11. inflammation around uterus ______
12. newborn ______
13. inflammation of vagina ______
14. no pregnancies ______
15. multiple births ______
16. blood in uterine tube ______
17. condition of no testes ______
18. pertaining to prostate ______
19. pertaining to sperm ______
20. surgical repair of glans penis ______
21. male producing ______
22. pertaining to testes ______
23. condition of scanty sperm ______
24. pertaining to the seminal vesicle ______
25. pertaining to epididymis ______

QUIZ 10E

Abbreviations Quiz

Directions: Write the medical term for which each abbreviation stands.

1. AB ______
2. BSE ______
3. AI ______
4. Cx ______
5. EMB ______
6. ERT ______
7. FEKG ______
8. FHR ______
9. FTND ______
10. GYN ______
11. HDN ______
12. HRT ______
13. HSG ______
14. LBW ______
15. LMP ______
16. NB ______
17. PID ______
18. OCPs ______
19. OB ______
20. DRE ______
21. BPH ______
22. GC ______
23. GU ______
24. PSA ______
25. TUR ______

QUIZ 10F

Chapter Review

PART I: Multiple Choice

Directions: Circle the correct answer.

1. Which organ is *not* part of the female internal genitalia?
   - **a.** clitoris
   - **b.** uterus
   - **c.** uterine tube
   - **d.** cervix
2. The beginning of menstruation and the ability to reproduce is known as
   - **a.** puberty.
   - **b.** menopause.
   - **c.** gestation.
   - **d.** postpartum.
3. The medical term *abruptio placenta* means
   - **a.** termination of pregnancy before fetus is viable.
   - **b.** fallen uterus.
   - **c.** placenta has become placed in the lower part of the uterus.
   - **d.** placenta tears away from the uterine wall prematurely.
4. The pathological term for a benign growth or tumor in the uterus is
   - **a.** endometriosis.
   - **b.** endometritis.
   - **c.** fibroid tumor.
   - **d.** prolapsed uterus.
5. The surgical term *episiorrhaphy* is defined as
   - **a.** plastic repair of the vagina.
   - **b.** suture of the vulva.
   - **c.** suture of the perineum.
   - **d.** creation of an artifical opening in a uterine tube.
6. Another medical term for spontaneous abortion is
   - **a.** stillbirth.
   - **b.** tubal pregnancy.
   - **c.** abruptio placentae.
   - **d.** miscarriage.

7. The failure of the testes to descend into the scrotum before birth is known as
   - a. anorchism.
   - b. cryptorchidism.
   - c. phimosis.
   - d. hydrocele.
8. The male sterilization procedure whereby a segment of the vas deferens is removed is called a
   - a. vesiculectomy.
   - b. vasovasostomy.
   - c. vasectomy.
   - d. vasotomy.
9. The medical term for surgical removal of the testicles in the male or the ovaries in the female is
   - a. castration.
   - b. cauterization.
   - c. circumcision.
   - d. sterilization.
10. An accumulation of fluid around the testes is called
   - a. testicular torsion.
   - b. hydrocele.
   - c. phimosis.
   - d. varicocele.

PART II: Matching

Directions: Match the term with its definition.

_____	**1.** OCPs	**a.** Delivery of infant through abdominal incision
_____	**2.** episiotomy	**b.** Destroys sperm
_____	**3.** cesarean section	**c.** Enlarged veins in spermatic cord
_____	**4.** chorionic villus sampling	**d.** Incision that facilitates birth process
_____	**5.** placenta previa	**e.** An STD
_____	**6.** meconium	**f.** Placenta blocks the birth canal
_____	**7.** spermatocide	**g.** Impotence
_____	**8.** genital warts	**h.** Birth control pills
_____	**9.** varicocele	**i.** Newborn's first bowel movement
_____	**10.** ED	**j.** Early test for genetic birth defects

PART III: Abbreviations

Directions: Write the full meaning of the following abbreviations.

1. ED ______________________________
2. TURP ______________________________
3. HPV ______________________________
4. FHR ______________________________
5. EMB ______________________________

Chapter 11

Endocrine System

Learning Objectives

Upon completion of this chapter, you will be able to:

- Identify and define the combining forms and suffixes introduced in this chapter.
- Correctly spell and pronounce medical terms and major anatomical structures relating to the endocrine system.
- Locate and describe the major organs of the endocrine system and their functions.
- List the major hormones secreted by each endocrine gland and describe their functions.
- Identify and define endocrine system anatomical terms.
- Identify and define selected endocrine system pathology terms.
- Identify and define selected endocrine system diagnostic procedures.
- Identify and define selected endocrine system therapeutic procedures.
- Identify and define selected medications relating to the endocrine system.
- Define selected abbreviations associated with the endocrine system.

WORKSHEET 11A

New Combining Form and Suffix

Directions: For each word part below, write its meaning. Then, locate a term from the chapter that uses the word part and its meaning.

Combining Forms	Meaning	Chapter Term	Meaning
1. acr/o	______	______	______
2. aden/o	______	______	______
3. adren/o	______	______	______
4. adrenal/o	______	______	______
5. andr/o	______	______	______
6. calc/o	______	______	______
7. crin/o	______	______	______
8. estr/o	______	______	______
9. gluc/o	______	______	______
10. glyc/o	______	______	______
11. gonad/o	______	______	______
12. iod/o	______	______	______
13. kal/i	______	______	______
14. ket/o	______	______	______
15. mineral/o	______	______	______
16. natr/o	______	______	______
17. ovari/o	______	______	______
18. pancreat/o	______	______	______
19. parathyroid/o	______	______	______
20. pineal/o	______	______	______
21. pituitar/o	______	______	______
22. radi/o	______	______	______
23. somat/o	______	______	______
24. testicul/o	______	______	______

25. thym/o ______________ ______________ ______________

26. thyr/o ______________ ______________ ______________

27. thyroid/o ______________ ______________ ______________

28. toxic/o ______________ ______________ ______________

Suffixes

29. -dipsia ______________ ______________ ______________

30. -emic ______________ ______________ ______________

31. -tropic ______________ ______________ ______________

32. -tropin ______________ ______________ ______________

WORKSHEET 11B

Medical Term Analysis

Directions: Below are terms built from word parts used in this and previous chapters. Analyze each term presented below, and list and define the word parts used to build each term.

Medical Term	**Word Part Analysis**
1. endocrine	________
2. homeostasis	________
3. androgen	________
4. estrogen	________
5. adrenocorticotropic	________
6. gonadotropin	________
7. somatotropin	________
8. endocrinology	________
9. gynecomastia	________
10. retinopathy	________
11. neuropathy	________
12. acromegaly	________
13. panhypopituitarism	________
14. thyrotoxicosis	________
15. adenocarcinoma	________
16. postprandial	________
17. lobectomy	________

WORKSHEET 11C

Unscramble

Directions: Unscramble each medical term below. A definition for the term is given below each scrambled term.

1. e n a t t y ____________________

   Nerve irritability and muscle cramps from hypocalcemia

2. a m i d r i o m o a n s a u s y ____________________

   Measures levels of hormones in blood plasma

3. y m d e a m x e ____________________

   Results from hyposecretion of thyroid hormones in an adult

4. a h s m s t i h o o ____________________

   Autoimmune form of thyroiditis

5. r e i g t o ____________________

   Enlarged thyroid gland

6. h p x h o t a e l o s m ____________________

   Protruding eyeballs

7. w i r f a s m d ____________________

   Being excessively short in height

8. i h g s u n c s syndrome ____________________

   Results from hypersecretion of adrenal cortex hormones

9. adrenal z i f n e i a m i t n o ____________________

   Female secondary sexual characteristics in a male

10. y c r l o i s g u a ____________________

    Sugar in the urine

WORKSHEET 11D

Sound It Out

Directions: The following are some of the important terms from this chapter written as their phonetic spellings. Sound out each term and write it in the blank.

1. thigh-roh-MEG-ah-lee ______
2. ah-dree-noh-MEG-ah-lee ______
3. eks-off-THAL-muss ______
4. pair-ah-thigh-royd-EK-toh-mee ______
5. ak-roh-MEG-ah-lee ______
6. en-doh-krin-ALL-oh-jee ______
7. ah-dree-nal-EK-toh-mee ______
8. gly-kohs-YOO-ree-ah ______
9. GOY-ter ______
10. high-per-pih-TOO-ih-tuh-rizm ______
11. miks-eh-DEE-mah ______
12. high-poh-pair-ah-THIGH-royd-izm ______
13. JYE-gan-tizm ______
14. high-poh-THIGH-royd-izm ______
15. oh-VAIR-ee-an ______
16. high-per-gly-SEE-mee-ah ______
17. pan-kree-AT-ik ______
18. pin-ee-ah-LEK-toh-mee ______
19. pol-ee-DIP-see-ah ______
20. tess-TIK-yoo-lar ______
21. TET-ah-nee ______
22. thigh-MY-tis ______
23. ah-DREE-nal ______
24. thigh-royd-EK-toh-mee ______
25. thigh-roh-tok-sih-KOH-sis ______

WORKSHEET 11E

Word Search Puzzle

Directions: Find and circle the answer for each fill-in-the-blank question in the word search puzzle.

L	C	E	D	E	M	A	I	R	M	S	R	L	M	A	G
B	L	Z	Y	B	M	L	L	G	Y	D	Y	G	B	M	B
W	T	P	V	N	B	R	I	C	L	I	X	M	Z	O	Q
K	R	J	W	K	A	G	P	K	A	O	Q	E	L	T	M
P	R	P	Q	K	A	T	R	R	G	R	V	L	V	Y	R
L	O	C	Q	N	Z	V	E	H	E	E	T	L	R	C	H
M	F	L	T	Q	D	V	C	T	M	T	H	I	V	O	F
K	L	I	Y	G	T	P	Q	Q	O	S	W	T	W	M	Z
R	S	N	N	D	L	R	M	T	R	O	T	U	W	O	Z
M	Y	B	Z	S	I	S	D	F	C	C	K	S	B	R	J
J	G	N	M	H	I	P	M	L	A	I	T	C	M	H	C
G	J	Z	G	L	V	P	S	H	M	T	R	V	W	C	L
Z	T	G	I	N	L	L	I	I	V	R	E	T	I	O	G
D	V	R	V	G	R	R	L	D	A	O	D	Q	M	E	T
Z	I	P	M	Y	Z	T	W	M	U	C	N	L	Q	H	M
V	J	M	B	R	T	Q	R	V	P	S	X	H	K	P	R

1. ____________________ results in the enlargement of bones of the head and extremities.
2. Adrenal ______________________________ is the appearance of male secondary sexual characteristics in a female.
3. ______________________________ are hormones with a strong anti-inflammatory action.
4. A condition in which body tissues contain excessive amounts of fluid is ________________.
5. Diabetes ____________________________ is caused by insufficient antidiuretic hormone whereas diabetesis a disorder of sugar metabolism.
6. Hypersecretion of growth hormone in a child or teenager results in ________________.
7. A(n) ____ is an enlarged thyroid gland.
8. __________________ is nerve irritability and painful muscle cramps from hypocalcemia.
9. __________________________________ is usually a benign tumor of the adrenal medulla.
10. ____ is a term meaning "excessive thirst."

WORKSHEET 11F

Crossword Puzzle

Directions: Use the definitions to complete the crossword puzzles.

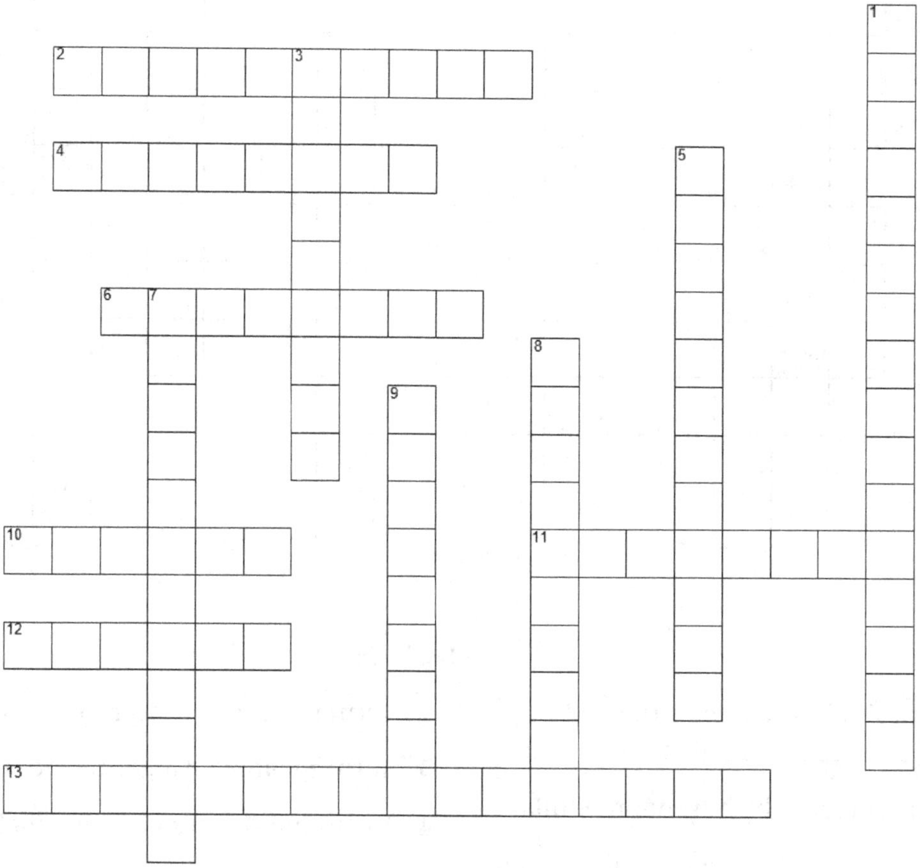

ACROSS

2 Term meaning "excessive thirst"

4 Hormone secreted by thymus gland

6 Diabetes ______________, one cause of insufficient insulin

10 Enlarged thyroid gland

11 Condition with swollen facial features and puffy, dry skin

12 Nerve irritability and painful muscle cramps

13 Usually benign tumor of adrenal medulla

DOWN

1 Test that measures level of hormones in blood

3 Diabetes ______________, caused by insufficient antidiuretic hormone

5 Term meaning "insufficient blood sugar level"

7 Protruding eyeballs

8 Excessive growth of bones of head and extremities

9 Excessive growth of entire body

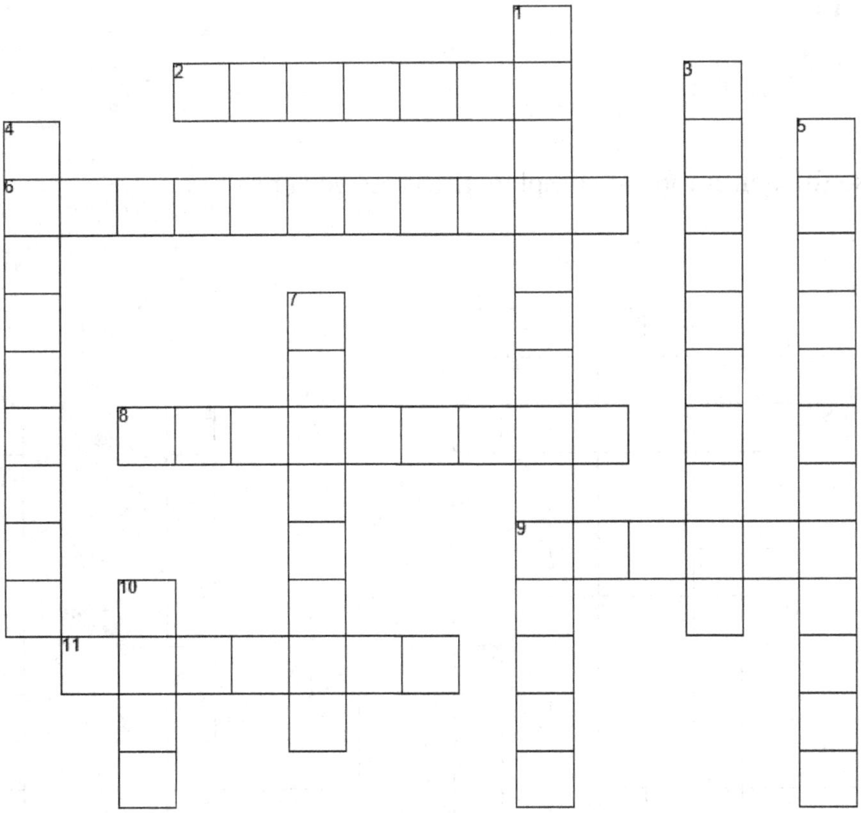

ACROSS

2 Hashimoto's disease affects the ____________________ gland

6 Hormone secreted by adrenal medulla

8 ____________________ gland, also called master gland

9 A thyroid scan uses radioactive

11 Chemical messenger secreted by endocrine glands

DOWN

1 Term meaning "cancerous tumor of a gland"

3 Term meaning "sugar in the urine"

4 Hormone secreted by pineal gland

5 Male sex hormone

7 Pancreas secretes insulin and ____________________

10 Number of parathyroid glands

WORKSHEET 11G

Chapter Review

Anatomy and Physiology

Directions: Fill in the blanks with the requested information.

1. The endocrine system is a collection of ____________________ that secrete ____________________ directly into the bloodstream.
2. The adrenal glands are located directly above the ____________________ and are divided into a ____________________ and ____________________.
3. The female gonad is the ________________, and the male gonad is the ________________.
4. The ____________________ is the only endocrine gland that is both an exocrine and endocrine gland.
5. Parathyroid hormone is responsible for regulating the level of ____________________ in the bloodstream.
6. ____________________ from the pineal gland is responsible for regulating circadian rhythm.
7. Prolactin stimulates ____________________ production by the ____________________.
8. Follicle-stimulating hormone and luteinizing hormone are collectively referred to as ____________________.
9. Antidiuretic hormone and oxytocin are secreted by the ____________________.
10. Thyroid gland hormones are produced using the mineral ____________________.

Word Building

Directions: Build a term for each of the following items.

1. adrenal gland disease ______
2. excessive calcium in the blood ______
3. low sugar in the blood ______
4. state of excessive parathyroid ______
5. pertaining to the pancreas ______
6. thymus tumor ______
7. state of insufficient thyroid ______
8. sugar in the urine ______
9. many (excessive) thirst ______
10. enlarged thyroid ______

Matching

Directions: Match the term with its definition.

_____ **1.** edema
_____ **2.** exophthalmos
_____ **3.** gynecomastia
_____ **4.** hirsutism
_____ **5.** syndrome
_____ **6.** virilism
_____ **7.** pheochromocytoma
_____ **8.** acidosis
_____ **9.** diabetes mellitus
_____ **10.** IDDM
_____ **11.** insulinoma
_____ **12.** tetany
_____ **13.** acromegaly
_____ **14.** dwarfism
_____ **15.** goiter
_____ **16.** Hashimoto's disease
_____ **17.** thyrotoxicosis
_____ **18.** FBS
_____ **19.** radioimmunoassay
_____ **20.** thyroid echography
_____ **21.** thyroid scan
_____ **22.** aquaretics
_____ **23.** hyperkalemia
_____ **24.** GH
_____ **25.** Exocrine

a. Tumor of adrenal medulla
b. Secrete into a duct
c. Type 1 diabetes mellitus
d. A pituitary gland hormone
e. Breast development in a male
f. Enlarged thyroid gland
g. Tumor of islets of Langerhans
h. Test using radioactive iodine
i. Tissues contain excessive amount of fluid
j. Short stature
k. Lab test for sugar level of blood
l. Development of male sex characteristics
m. Bulging eyeballs
n. Marked overproduction of thyroid hormones
o. Enlargement of bones of extremities
p. Measures levels of hormones in the blood
q. Excessive amount of hair
r. An ultrasound examination
s. Nerve irritability
t. Increases water secretion by kidney
u. Group of symptoms occurring together
v. Autoimmune form of thyroiditis
w. Symptoms are hyperglycemia and glycosuria
x. Too much potassium in the blood
y. Excess acid in the body tissues

QUIZ 11A

New Word Parts Quiz

Directions: Define the combining form or suffix in the spaces provided.

1. acr/o ______________________________
2. adren/o ______________________________
3. radi/o ______________________________
4. calc/o ______________________________
5. crin/o ______________________________
6. somat/o ______________________________
7. gonad/o ______________________________
8. kal/i ______________________________
9. natr/o ______________________________
10. aden/o ______________________________
11. pancreat/o ______________________________
12. parathyroid/o ______________________________
13. pineal/o ______________________________
14. pituitar/o ______________________________
15. thym/o ______________________________
16. adrenal/o ______________________________
17. thyr/o ______________________________
18. toxic/o ______________________________
19. glyc/o ______________________________
20. testicul/o ______________________________
21. iod/o ______________________________
22. -dipsia ______________________________
23. -emic ______________________________
24. -tropic ______________________________
25. -tropin ______________________________

QUIZ 11B

Labeling Diagram

Directions: Label the structures in the diagram.

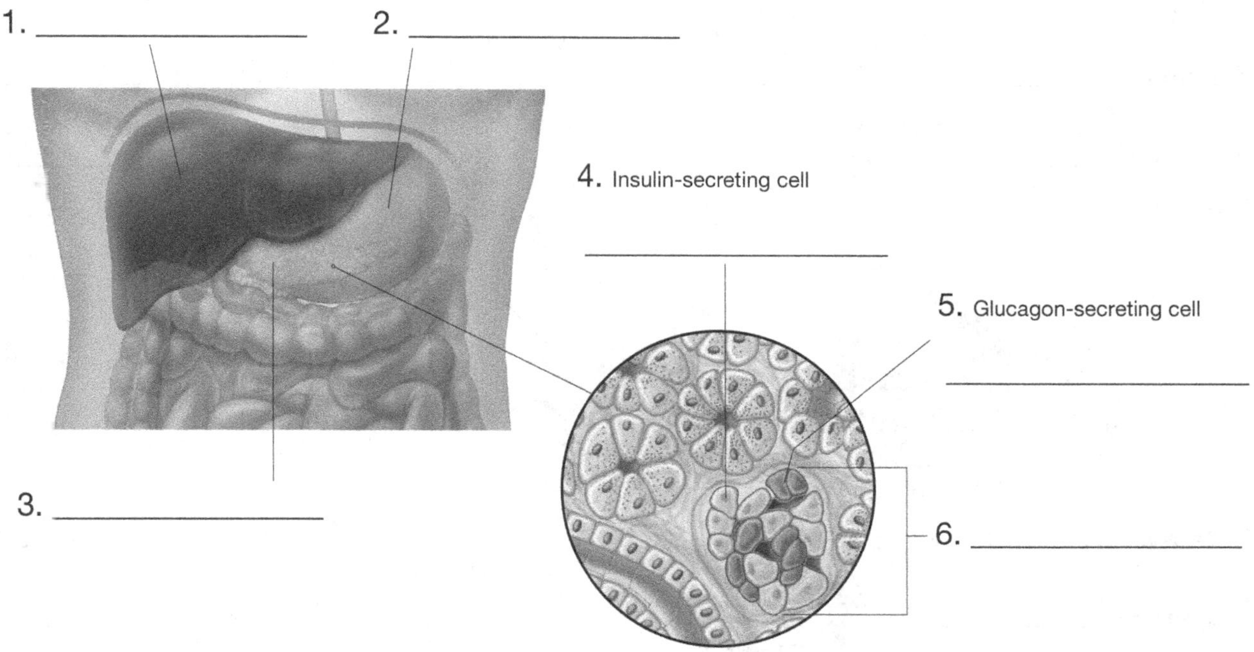

QUIZ 11C

Labeling Diagram

Directions: Label the hormones and target organs of the anterior pituitary gland.

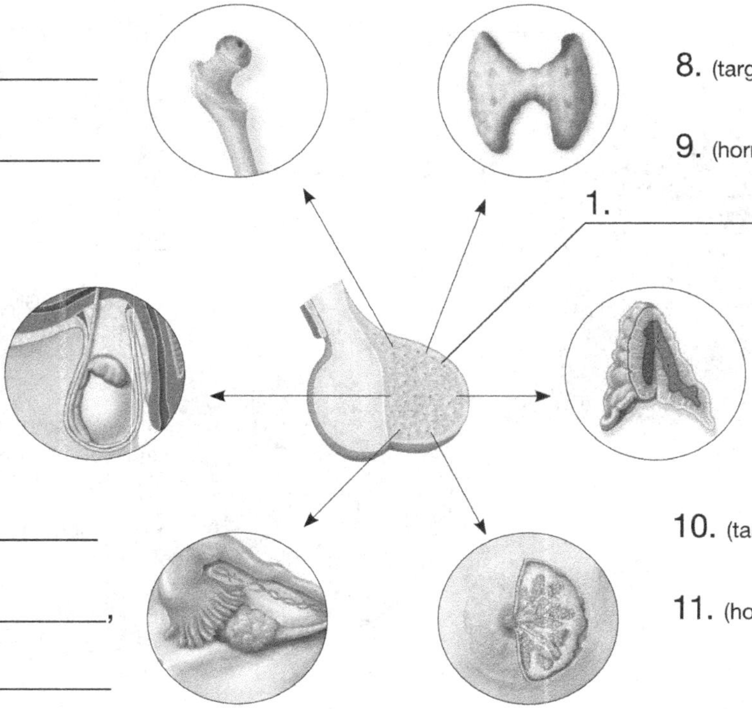

1. ________________

2. (target)________________

3. (hormone)________________

8. (target)________________

9. (hormone)________________

4. (target)________________

5. (hormones)________________, ________________

10. (target)________________

11. (hormone)________________

6. (target)________________

7. (hormones)________________, ________________

12. (target)________________

13. (hormone)________________

QUIZ 11D

Word Building Quiz

Directions: Build a single medical term for each phrase below.

1. thymus inflammation ______
2. pertaining to the parathyroid gland ______
3. pertaining to the pancreas ______
4. pertaining to the thymus gland ______
5. pertaining to the thyroid gland ______
6. removal of the thyroid ______
7. state of insufficient pituitary ______
8. low sodium in the blood ______
9. excessive potassium in the blood ______
10. specialist in the endocrine system ______
11. excessive calcium in the blood ______
12. low sugar in the blood ______
13. adrenal gland disease ______
14. enlarged extremities ______
15. condition of too much urine ______

QUIZ 11E

Abbreviations Quiz

Directions: Write the medical term for which each abbreviation stands.

1. ACTH ______________________________
2. ADH ______________________________
3. BMR ______________________________
4. DI ______________________________
5. DM ______________________________
6. FBS ______________________________
7. FSH ______________________________
8. GH ______________________________
9. GTT ______________________________
10. IDDM ______________________________
11. K+ ______________________________
12. Na+ ______________________________
13. CT ______________________________
14. PBI ______________________________
15. PRL ______________________________
16. PTH ______________________________
17. RIA ______________________________
18. T3 ______________________________
19. T4 ______________________________
20. TFT ______________________________
21. TSH ______________________________
22. NIDDM ______________________________
23. NPH ______________________________
24. LH ______________________________
25. MSH ______________________________

QUIZ 11F

Chapter Review

Directions: Circle the correct answer.

1. The hormone that aids the body in regulating carbohydrates is
   - **a.** cortisol.
   - **b.** epinephrine.
   - **c.** aldosterone.
   - **d.** oxytocin.
2. Which of the following is *not* an endocrine gland?
   - **a.** thyroid
   - **b.** pancreas
   - **c.** pituitary
   - **d.** lacrimal
3. Which hormone is *not* secreted by the anterior lobe of the pituitary gland?
   - **a.** prolactin
   - **b.** antidiuretic hormone
   - **c.** thyroid-stimulating hormone
   - **d.** growth hormone
4. Insulin-dependent diabetes mellitus is also known as
   - **a.** type 1.
   - **b.** Recklinghausen disease.
   - **c.** type 2.
   - **d.** myxedema.
5. The term *hyperkalemia* is defined as
   - **a.** excess potassium in the blood.
   - **b.** excess sugar in the blood.
   - **c.** excess sodium in the blood.
   - **d.** excess calcium in the blood.
6. The term for a condition of painful muscle cramps resulting from a low amount of calcium in the blood is
   - **a.** myxedema.
   - **b.** tetany.
   - **c.** goiter.
   - **d.** acidosis.
7. The term for the condition of having an excessive amount of hair is
   - **a.** exophthalmos.
   - **b.** syndrome.
   - **c.** gynecomastia.
   - **d.** hirsutism.
8. Thyroid function tests are
   - **a.** tests in which a radioactive element is administered.
   - **b.** blood test used to measure the levels of T3, T4, and TSH.
   - **c.** ultrasound examination of the thyroid.
   - **d.** procedure where the thyroid is destroyed.

9. The disease resulting from hypersecretion by the adrenal cortex is

a. Addison's disease.

b. Graves' disease.

c. Cushing's syndrome.

d. Hashimoto's thyroiditis.

10. Goiter is enlargement of the

a. adrenal glands.

b. pituitary gland.

c. parathyroid glands.

d. thyroid gland.

PART II: Matching

Directions: Match the term with its definition.

_____ **1.** growth hormone	**a.** Test for thyroid function
_____ **2.** hormone replacement therapy	**b.** Excess body fluids
_____ **3.** protein-bound iodine test	**c.** May result in blindness
_____ **4.** myxedema	**d.** Secreted by the pancreas
_____ **5.** diabetic retinopathy	**e.** Caused by inadequate secretion of ADH
_____ **6.** gynecomastia	**f.** Treats children with abnormal short stature
_____ **7.** edema	**g.** Secreted by the posterior pituitary gland
_____ **8.** glucagon	**h.** Hyposecretion of thyroid in adults
_____ **9.** antidiuretic hormone	**i.** Symptom of adrenal feminization
_____ **10.** diabetes insipidus	**j.** Treatment for hyposecretion disorders

PART III: Abbreviations

Directions: Write the full meaning of the following abbreviations.

1. IDDM ____________________

2. PBI ____________________

3. FBS ____________________

4. Na^+ ____________________

5. T_4 ____________________

Chapter 12

Nervous System and Mental Health

Learning Objectives

Upon completion of this chapter, you will be able to:

- Identify and define the combining forms and suffixes introduced in this chapter.
- Correctly spell and pronounce medical terms and major anatomical structures relating to the nervous system.
- Locate and describe the major organs of the nervous system and their functions.
- Describe the components of a neuron.
- Distinguish between the central nervous system, peripheral nervous system, and autonomic nervous system.
- Identify and define nervous system anatomical terms.
- Identify and define selected nervous system pathology terms.
- Identify and define selected nervous system diagnostic procedures.
- Identify and define selected nervous system therapeutic procedures.
- Identify and define selected medications relating to the nervous system.
- Define selected abbreviations associated with the nervous system.
- Describe examples of each classification of mental disorders.
- Identify and define selected mental health therapeutic procedures.
- Define selected abbreviations associated with mental health.

WORKSHEET 12A

New Combining Form and Suffix

Directions: For each word part below, write its meaning. Then, locate a term from the chapter that uses the word part and its meaning.

Combining Forms	Meaning	Chapter Term	Meaning
1. alges/o	______	______	______
2. astr/o	______	______	______
3. centr/o	______	______	______
4. cerebell/o	______	______	______
5. cerebr/o	______	______	______
6. clon/o	______	______	______
7. concuss/o	______	______	______
8. dur/o	______	______	______
9. encephal/o	______	______	______
10. esthesi/o	______	______	______
11. gli/o	______	______	______
12. medull/o	______	______	______
13. mening/o	______	______	______
14. meningi/o	______	______	______
15. ment/o	______	______	______
16. myel/o	______	______	______
17. neur/o	______	______	______
18. peripher/o	______	______	______
19. poli/o	______	______	______
20. pont/o	______	______	______
21. radicul/o	______	______	______
22. thalam/o	______	______	______

23. thec/o ______ ______ ______
24. tom/o ______ ______ ______
25. ton/o ______ ______ ______
26. ventricul/o ______ ______ ______
27. amnes/o ______ ______ ______
28. anxi/o ______ ______ ______
29. compuls/o ______ ______ ______
30. delus/o ______ ______ ______
31. depress/o ______ ______ ______
32. electr/o ______ ______ ______
33. hallucin/o ______ ______ ______
34. klept/o ______ ______ ______
35. ment/o ______ ______ ______
36. narc/o ______ ______ ______
37. neur/o ______ ______ ______
38. obsess/o ______ ______ ______
39. ped/o ______ ______ ______
40. pharmac/o ______ ______ ______
41. phob/o ______ ______ ______
42. phren/o ______ ______ ______
43. psych/o ______ ______ ______
44. pyr/o ______ ______ ______
45. schiz/o ______ ______ ______
46. soci/o ______ ______ ______
47. somat/o ______ ______ ______
48. somn/o ______ ______ ______
49. vers/o ______ ______ ______

Suffixes

50. –paresis ______ ______ ______
51. –phasia ______ ______ ______
52. –taxia ______ ______ ______
53. –iatric ______ ______ ______
54. –iatrist ______ ______ ______
55. –iatry ______ ______ ______
56. –lepsy ______ ______ ______
57. –logist ______ ______ ______
58. –mania ______ ______ ______
59. –orexia ______ ______ ______
60. –philic ______ ______ ______
61. –phoria ______ ______ ______
62. – therapy ______ ______ ______

WORKSHEET 12B

Medical Term Analysis

Directions: Below are terms built from word parts used in this and previous chapters. Analyze each term presented below, and list and define the word parts used to build each term.

Medical Term	**Word Part Analysis**
1. cranial	______________________________
2. neuroglial	______________________________
3. somatic	______________________________
4. anesthesiology	______________________________
5. hemiparesis	______________________________
6. hemiplegia	______________________________
7. neurology	______________________________
8. amyotrophic	______________________________
9. meningocele	______________________________
10. myelomeningocele	______________________________
11. poliomyelitis	______________________________
12. schizophrenia	______________________________
13. kleptomania	______________________________
14. electroencephalography	______________________________
15. analgesic	______________________________

WORKSHEET 12C

Unscramble

Directions: Unscramble each medical term below. A definition for the term is given below each scrambled term.

1. s e i p l e p y ______________________________

   Seizures and loss of consciousness due to uncontrolled neuron electrical activity

2. n u c n u o s i o c s ______________________________

   Being unaware of surroundings; does not respond to stimuli

3. i n t c n v u a l o n a t s ______________________________

   Medication to control seizures

4. n e i l n m o e c g e ______________________________

   Protrusion of the meninges

5. l a l u i c n h n a i o t ______________________________

   Perceiving something that is not there

6. r o h e c h p y a s l u d ______________________________

   Accumulation of cerebrospinal fluid in brain ventricles

7. o l p e y n i u r i s t ______________________________

   Inflammation of many nerves

8. s n i a o n i m ______________________________

   Inability to sleep

9. e h p m i g l i e a ______________________________

   Paralysis of half the body

10. h a p i a s a ______________________________

    Unable to speak

WORKSHEET 12D

Sound It Out

Directions: The following are some of the important terms from this chapter written as their phonetic spellings. Sound out each term and write it in the blank.

1. men-in-JYE-tis ____________________
2. noo-ROH-mah ____________________
3. sair-eh-BELL-ar ____________________
4. kon-KUSH-un ____________________
5. en-seff-ah-LYE-tis ____________________
6. deh-MEN-sha ____________________
7. an-es-THEE-zha ____________________
8. dis-FAY-zee-ah ____________________
9. en-seh-FAL-ik ____________________
10. noo-REK-toh-mee ____________________
11. sigh-KIGH-ah-tree ____________________
12. hem-ee-PLEE-jee-ah ____________________
13. high-droh-SEFF-ah-lus ____________________
14. meh-NIN-jee-all ____________________
15. thah-LAM-ik ____________________
16. AW-tizm ____________________
17. noo-RALL-oh-jee ____________________
18. my-eh-LOG-rah-fee ____________________
19. noo-RAL-jee-ah ____________________
20. NOOR-oh-plas-tee ____________________
21. pah-RAL-ih-sis ____________________
22. my-eh-LYE-tis ____________________
23. SEE-zyoor ____________________
24. seh-ree-broh-VAS-kyoo-lar ____________________
25. SIN-koh-pee ____________________

WORKSHEET 12E

Word Search Puzzle

Directions: Find and circle the answer for each fill-in-the-blank question in the word search puzzle.

W	D	M	N	T	F	N	E	C	D	Z	M	P	V
K	L	H	T	F	M	P	R	E	S	T	B	L	D
S	K	B	H	P	O	Q	M	B	R	G	C	H	L
I	S	N	H	C	A	E	B	N	E	M	G	W	T
S	L	I	N	K	N	L	O	F	M	H	P	M	H
Y	R	Y	S	T	K	I	S	N	I	R	N	M	G
L	S	Q	I	O	S	H	H	Y	E	F	Y	T	N
A	Z	A	J	U	R	R	C	K	H	N	J	M	K
R	Z	B	T	K	L	E	R	X	Z	J	C	Z	K
A	N	N	T	L	Z	L	L	J	L	N	O	N	L
P	O	T	F	L	N	W	P	C	A	G	M	J	L
C	G	Z	Q	R	G	K	W	K	S	M	A	H	L
A	N	T	I	C	O	N	V	U	L	S	A	N	T
S	U	L	A	H	P	E	C	O	R	D	Y	H	R

1. ______________________ disease is a chronic condition with progressive disorientation and loss of memory.
2. ____________________________ medication reduces excitability of neurons to prevent uncontrolled neuron activity.
3. Cerebral ____________________________ is the bruising of the brain from impact, with symptoms lasting longer than 24 hours.
4. Cerebral ____________________________ is brain damage resulting from a defect in fetal development or oxygen deprivation at time of birth.
5. The state of profound unconsciousness is called ____________________________.

6. Progressive impairment of intellectual function interfering with performing daily activities is called ______________________________.

7. ____ results from the buildup of cerebrospinal fluid.

8. Multiple __________________________________ is an autoimmune disease affecting the central nervous system.

9. ____ is the loss of muscle function and movement.

10. The medical term for fainting is ____.

WORKSHEET 12F

Crossword Puzzle

Directions: Use the definitions to complete the crossword puzzles.

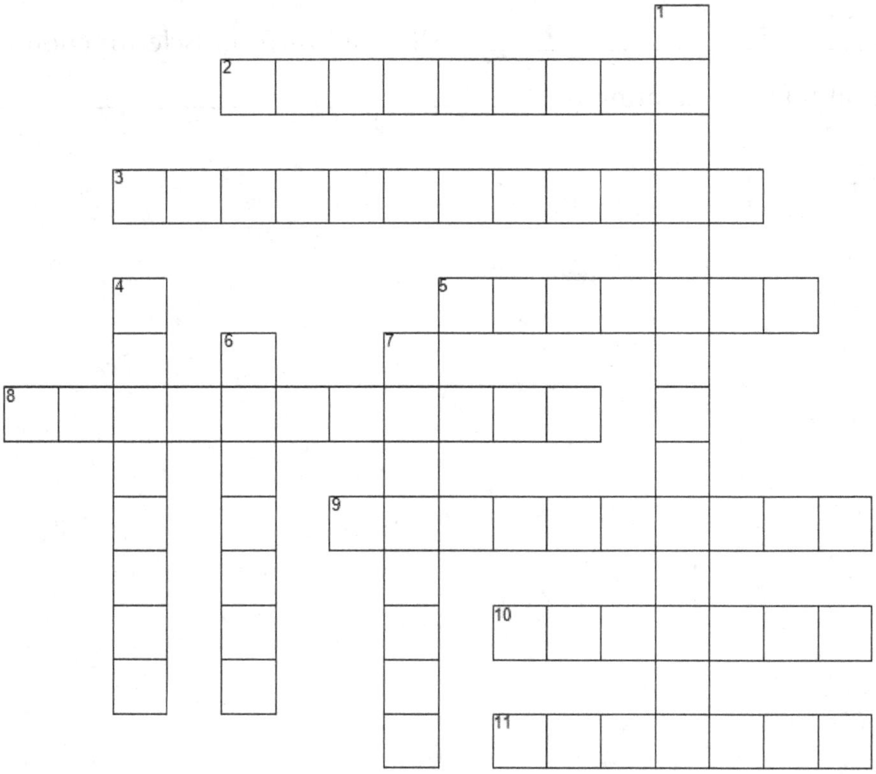

ACROSS

2 Cerebral ______________________, bruising of the brain

3 Term meaning "paralysis of four (limbs)"

5 ______________________ nerves carry information to the CNS

8 Muscle weakness in one limb

9 Coordinates body movement and maintains balance

10 Point where one neuron meets another

11 The brain and spinal cord form the ______________________ nervous system

DOWN

1 Medication that reduces neuron excitability

4 Protective covering around the brain and spinal cord

6 Term meaning "without speech"

7 Largest part of the brain

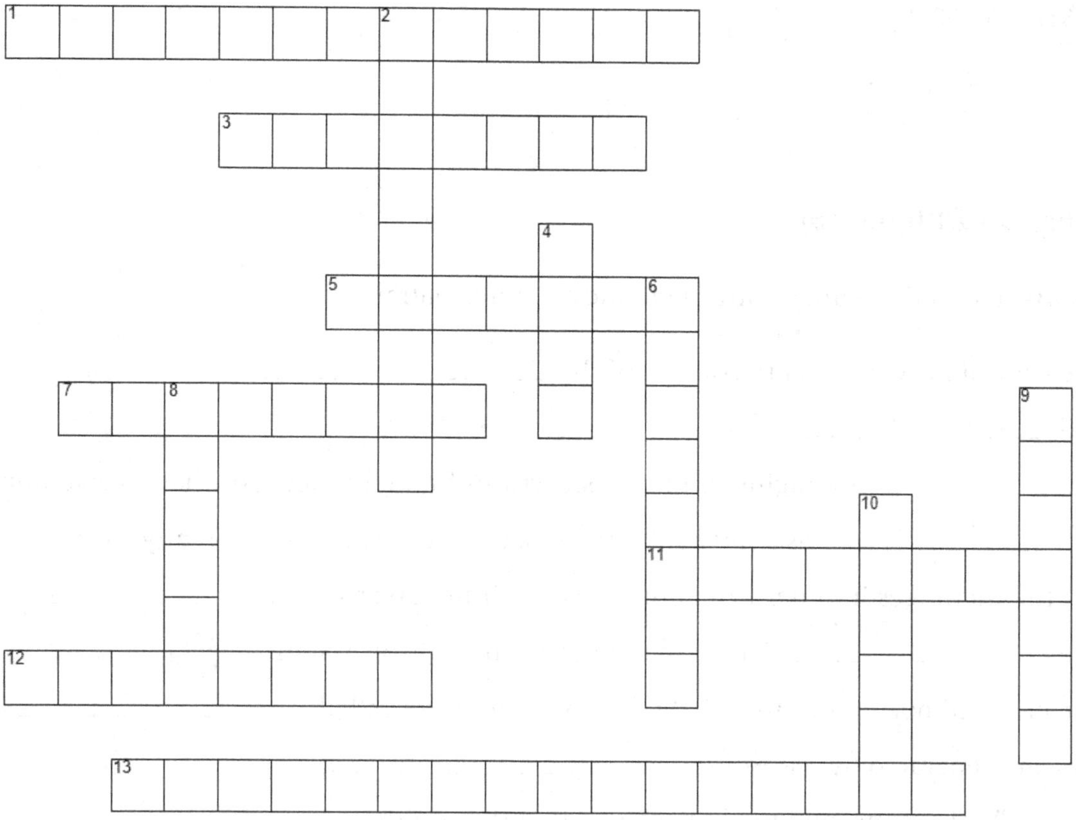

ACROSS

1 Buildup of cerebrospinal fluid within the brain

3 Headache with severe pain, dizziness, and nausea

5 Fainting

7 Progressive impairment of intellectual function

11 A PET scan uses ______________ radionuclides

12 Condition with painful blisters along nerve path

13 Myasthenia gravis happens because of insufficient ______________

DOWN

2 The temporary or permanent loss of muscle function

4 Profound unconsciousness

6 Seizures caused by uncontrolled neuron electrical activity

8 In multiple sclerosis, the immune system destroys ______________

9 Petit mal is also called a(n) ______________ seizure

10 Common name for cerebrovascular accident

WORKSHEET 12G

Chapter Review

Anatomy and Physiology

Directions: Fill in the blanks with the requested information.

1. The central nervous system consists of the ____________________ and ____________________.
2. ________________ are highly branched structures found on neurons that receive impulses.
3. ____________________ is a fatty substance that acts as insulation for many axons.
4. List the meninges in order from outer layer to inner layer: ____________________.
5. The ____________________ lobe of the cerebrum controls vision.
6. The elevated portions of the cerebral convolutions are called ____________________ and they are separated by fissures called ____________________.
7. The midbrain, pons, and medulla oblongata make up the ____________________.
8. Pain perception is controlled by the ____________________.
9. The point at which a nerve is attached to the central nervous system is called the ____________________.
10. The ____________________ branch of the ANS is the "fight-or-flight" branch and the ____________________ branch of the ANS is the "rest-and-digest" branch.

Word Building

Directions: Build a term for each of the following items.

1. brain inflammation ____________________
2. head pain ____________________
3. pertaining to the cerebrum and spine ____________________
4. tumor of the meninges ____________________
5. surgical repair of nerve ____________________
6. absence of pain ____________________
7. without appetite ____________________
8. paralysis of four ____________________
9. lack of muscle coordination ____________________
10. sleep seizure ____________________

Matching

Directions: Match the term with its definition.

____ **1.** absence seizure
____ **2.** aura
____ **3.** DSM
____ **4.** delirium
____ **5.** focal seizure
____ **6.** dementia
____ **7.** paresthesia
____ **8.** syncope
____ **9.** tremor
____ **10.** unconscious
____ **11.** astrocytoma
____ **12.** cerebral aneurysm
____ **13.** cerebral contusion
____ **14.** CVA
____ **15.** Reye syndrome
____ **16.** enuresis
____ **17.** ALS
____ **18.** spina bifida
____ **19.** MS
____ **20.** myasthenia gravis
____ **21.** brain scan
____ **22.** lumbar puncture
____ **23.** laminectomy
____ **24.** anticonvulsant
____ **25.** hypnotic

a. Voiding urine in inappropriate places
b. Confusion, disorientation, agitation
c. Procedure removes pressure on spinal nerve
d. Repetitive, alternating movements
e. Controls seizures
f. Unaware of surroundings
g. Insufficient neurotransmitter
h. Petit mal
i. Associated with children taking aspirin
j. Bruising of the brain
k. A stroke
l. Manual that organizes mental disorders into categories
m. Progressive spinal cord degeneration
n. Fainting
o. Impaired intellectual functioning
p. Nerves lose myelin sheath
q. Brain image made using radioactive isotopes
r. Unusual sensation before a seizure or migraine
s. Spinal tap
t. Burning or tingling sensations
u. Promotes sleep
v. May cause a hemorrhagic stroke
w. Affects only one limb
x. Congenital defect
y. Tumor of a neuroglial cell

QUIZ 12A

New Word Parts Quiz

Directions: Define the combining form or suffix in the spaces provided.

1. concuss/o ______
2. cerebell/o ______
3. cerebr/o ______
4. encephal/o ______
5. gli/o ______
6. mening/o ______
7. myel/o ______
8. neur/o ______
9. astr/o ______
10. poli/o ______
11. pont/o ______
12. radicul/o ______
13. thalam/o ______
14. ventricul/o ______
15. medull/o ______
16. esthesi/o ______
17. -paresis ______
18. -taxia ______
19. compuls/o ______
20. depress/o ______
21. narc/o ______
22. ped/o ______
23. pyr/o ______
24. -lepsy ______
25. -mania ______

QUIZ 12B

Labeling Diagram

Directions: Label the components of a neuron.

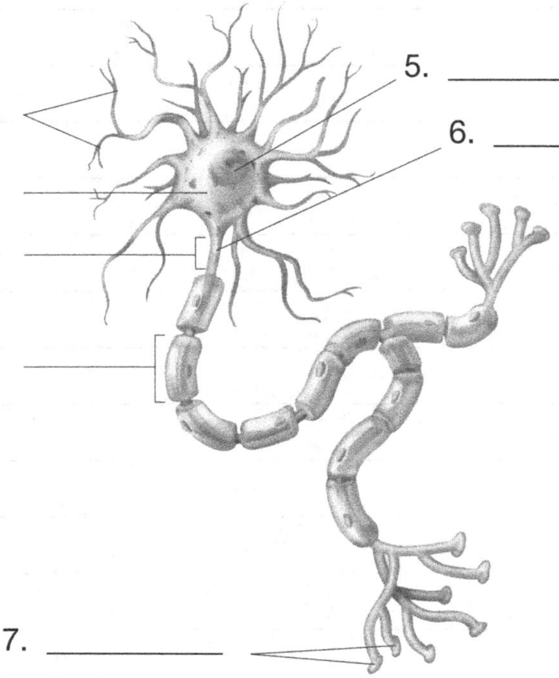

1. ____________
2. ____________
3. ____________
4. ____________
5. ____________
6. ____________
7. ____________

QUIZ 12C

Labeling Diagram

Directions: Label the parts of the brain.

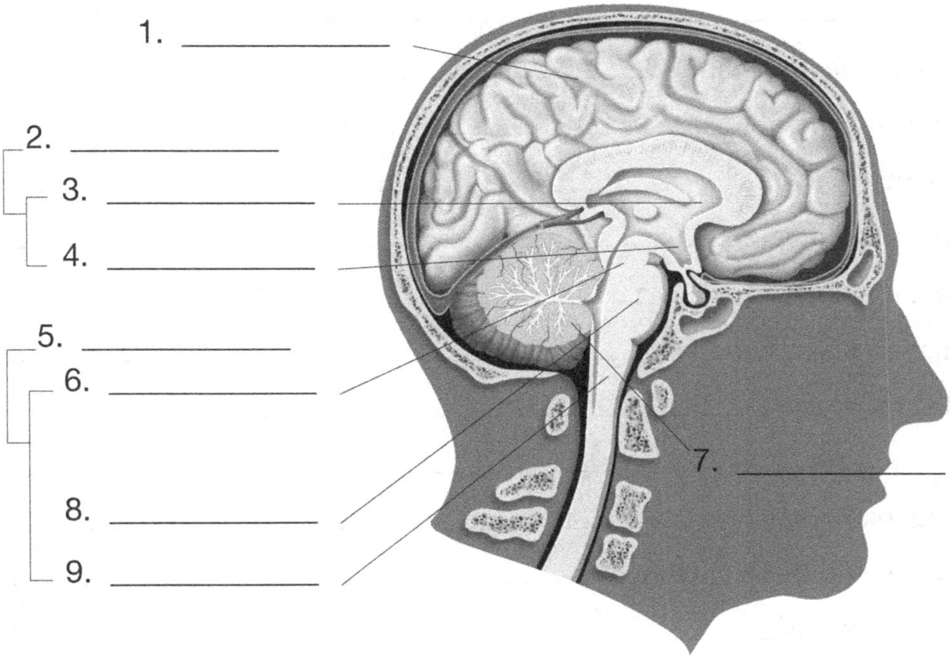

QUIZ 12D

Word Building Quiz

Directions: Build a single medical term for each phrase below.

1. head pain ______
2. pertaining to the cerebellum ______
3. irrational fear condition ______
4. record of brain's electricity ______
5. pertaining to meninges ______
6. pertaining to nerve ______
7. inflammation of many nerves ______
8. pertaining to the pons ______
9. nerve root disease ______
10. pertaining to the thalamus ______
11. pertaining to within the meninges ______
12. excessive sensations ______
13. forgetfulness condition ______
14. lack of speech ______
15. lack of muscle coordination ______
16. study of mind drugs ______
17. pertaining to the cerebrum and spine ______
18. half weakness ______
19. pertaining to nerve glue ______
20. surgical repair of a nerve ______

QUIZ 12E

Abbreviations Quiz

Directions: Write the medical term for which each abbreviation stands.

1. ALS ______________________________
2. ANS ______________________________
3. CNS ______________________________
4. CP ______________________________
5. CSF ______________________________
6. CVA ______________________________
7. CVD ______________________________
8. EEG ______________________________
9. ADHD ______________________________
10. ICP ______________________________
11. LP ______________________________
12. ECT ______________________________
13. PET ______________________________
14. BPD ______________________________
15. SCI ______________________________
16. TBI ______________________________
17. TIA ______________________________

QUIZ 12F

Chapter Review

PART I: Multiple Choice

Directions: Circle the correct answer.

1. The innermost layer of the meninges is the
   - **a.** arachnoid layer.
   - **b.** dura mater.
   - **c.** pia mater.
   - **d.** pons.
2. Afferent neurons
   - **a.** carry impulses to the brain and spinal cord.
   - **b.** carry impulses away from the brain and spinal cord.
   - **c.** carry impulses to the brain but away from the spinal cord.
   - **d.** carry impulses to the spinal cord but away from the brain.
3. The condition in which there is degeneration of the motor neurons of the spinal cord (Lou Gehrig's disease) is known as
   - **a.** myasthenia gravis.
   - **b.** multiple sclerosis.
   - **c.** amyotrophic lateral sclerosis.
   - **d.** Reye's syndrome.
4. One-sided facial paralysis with an unknown cause is known as
   - **a.** Reye's syndrome.
   - **b.** Lou Gehrig's disease.
   - **c.** Parkinson's disease.
   - **d.** Bell's palsy.
5. Amnesia and dissociative identity disorder are examples of
   - **a.** anxiety disorders.
   - **b.** impulse disorders.
   - **c.** mood disorders.
   - **d.** dissociative disorders.
6. The diagnostic term that means the process of x-ray filming the blood vessels of the brain is
   - **a.** cerebral angiogram.
   - **b.** ventriculogram.
   - **c.** myelography.
   - **d.** cerebral angiography.
7. The form of epilepsy in which there is a loss of awareness without muscle convulsions is
   - **a.** absence seizure.
   - **b.** palsy seizure.
   - **c.** focal seizure.
   - **d.** tonic-clonic seizure.

8. Which of the following is *not* a method of treating mental disorders?
   - a. psychopharmacology
   - b. electroconvulsive therapy
   - c. psychotherapy
   - d. phrenology
9. The condition characterized by nonprogressive paralysis from a defect or trauma at birth is
   - a. autism.
   - b. epilepsy.
   - c. cerebral palsy.
   - d. dementia.
10. The term for a disease affecting children and adolescents, typically following a viral infection, is
    - a. Babinski's syndrome.
    - b. cerebral palsy.
    - c. multiple sclerosis.
    - d. Reye's syndrome.

PART II: Matching

Directions: Match the term with its definition.

_____	**1.** cerebrospinal fluid shunt	**a.** Can pinpoint nerve damage
_____	**2.** nerve block	**b.** Progressive dementia
_____	**3.** nerve conduction velocity	**c.** Conducts electrical impulse on nerve
_____	**4.** subdural hematoma	**d.** Injection of regional anesthetic to stop pain
_____	**5.** shingles	**e.** Awake and aware of surroundings
_____	**6.** Alzheimer's disease	**f.** Binge eating and intentional vomiting
_____	**7.** conscious	**g.** Painful blisters along nerve path
_____	**8.** axon	**h.** Blood accumulating in meninges
_____	**9.** bulimia	**i.** Treats severe pain
_____	**10.** narcotic analgesic	**j.** Treats hydrocephalus

PART III: Abbreviations

Directions: Write the full meaning of the following abbreviations.

1. ANS ______________________________
2. CP ______________________________
3. SCI ______________________________
4. SAD ______________________________
5. MS ______________________________

Chapter 13

Special Senses: The Eye and Ear

Learning Objectives

Upon completion of this chapter, you will be able to:

- Identify and define the combining forms, suffixes, and prefixes introduced in this chapter.
- Correctly spell and pronounce medical terms and major anatomical structures relating to the eye and ear.
- Locate and describe the major structures of the eye and ear and their functions.
- Describe the process of vision.
- Describe the path of sound vibration.
- Identify and define eye and ear anatomical terms.
- Identify and define selected eye and ear pathology terms.
- Identify and define selected eye and ear diagnostic procedures.
- Identify and define selected eye and ear therapeutic procedures.
- Identify and define selected medications relating to the eye and ear.
- Define selected abbreviations associated with the eye and ear.

WORKSHEET 13A

New Combining Form and Suffix

Directions: For each word part below, write its meaning. Then, locate a term from the chapter that uses the word part and its meaning.

Combining Forms	Meaning	Chapter Term	Meaning
1. ambly/o			
2. aque/o			
3. blast/o			
4. blephar/o			
5. chromat/o			
6. conjunctiv/o			
7. corne/o			
8. cycl/o			
9. dacry/o			
10. dipl/o			
11. emmetr/o			
12. glauc/o			
13. ir/o			
14. irid/o			
15. kerat/o			
16. lacrim/o			
17. macul/o			
18. mi/o			
19. mydr/i			
20. nyctal/o			
21. ocul/o			
22. ophthalm/o			
23. opt/o			

24. optic/o ______ ______ ______

25. papill/o ______ ______ ______

26. phac/o ______ ______ ______

27. phot/o ______ ______ ______

28. presby/o ______ ______ ______

29. pupill/o ______ ______ ______

30. retin/o ______ ______ ______

31. scler/o ______ ______ ______

32. stigmat/o ______ ______ ______

33. uve/o ______ ______ ______

34. vitre/o ______ ______ ______

35. acous/o ______ ______ ______

36. audi/o ______ ______ ______

37. audit/o ______ ______ ______

38. aur/o ______ ______ ______

39. auricul/o ______ ______ ______

40. cerumin/o ______ ______ ______

41. cochle/o ______ ______ ______

42. labyrinth/o ______ ______ ______

43. mying/o ______ ______ ______

44. ot/o ______ ______ ______

45. salping/o ______ ______ ______

46. staped/o ______ ______ ______

47. tympan/o ______ ______ ______

48. vestibul/o ______ ______ ______

Suffixes

49. -ician ______ ______ ______

50. -metrist ______ ______ ______

51. -opia ______ ______ ______

52. -opsia ______ ______ ______

53. -phobia ______ ______ ______

54. -tropia ______ ______ ______

55. -cusis ______ ______ ______

56. -otia ______ ______ ______

Prefixes

57. eso- ______ ______ ______

58. exo- ______ ______ ______

59. myo- ______ ______ ______

WORKSHEET 13B

Medical Term Analysis

Directions: Below are terms built from word parts used in this and previous chapters. Analyze each term presented below, and list and define the word parts used to build each term.

Medical Term	Word Part Analysis
1. aqueous	____________________
2. vitreous	____________________
3. nyctalopia	____________________
4. optometry	____________________
5. presbyopia	____________________
6. amblyopia	____________________
7. monochromatism	____________________
8. exotropia	____________________
9. hemianopia	____________________
10. keratometry	____________________
11. ophthalmoscopy	____________________
12. cryoretinopexy	____________________
13. keratoplasty	____________________
14. otorhinolaryngology	____________________
15. presbycusis	____________________
16. ceruminoma	____________________
17. otosclerosis	____________________
18. labyrinthitis	____________________
19. otoscopy	____________________
20. tympanometry	____________________

WORKSHEET 13C

Scramble

Directions: Unscramble each medical term below. A definition for the term is given below each scrambled term.

1. t r a e t p a o l s k y ______________________

   Surgical repair of the cornea

2. m t a u g s n y s ______________________

   Jerky involuntary eye movements

3. p o y a m I ______________________

   Near-sightedness

4. a a a i o c h m p r s t ______________________

   Profound inability to see color

5. a e u u o s q ______________________

   Pertaining to water

6. p o n c i i t a ______________________

   Healthcare professional trained to make corrective lenses

7. a t s r s i b s u m ______________________

   Weakness of external eye muscles

8. l u c o c o m i o s s y ______________________

   Fungus infection of the eye

9. x m a p o t r h e n r i s y ______________________

   Term meaning "ruptured eardrum"

10. s i n t t i u n ______________________

    Ringing in the ears

WORKSHEET 13D

Sound It Out

Directions: The following are some of the important terms from this chapter written as their phonetic spellings. Sound out each term and write it in the blank.

1. off-THAL-mik ______
2. KAIR-ah-toh-plass-tee ______
3. RET-in-al ______
4. kon-junk-tih-VYE-tis ______
5. op-TOM-eh-trist ______
6. glau-KOH-mah ______
7. hem-ee-ah-NOP-ee-ah ______
8. ah-STIG-mah-tizm ______
9. in-trah-OCK-yoo-lar ______
10. LAK-rim-al ______
11. my-OH-pee-ah ______
12. KAT-ah-rakt ______
13. PYOO-pih-lair-ee ______
14. KOR-nee-all ______
15. foh-toh-FOH-bee-ah ______
16. KOK-lee-ar ______
17. OH-toh-plas-tee ______
18. AW-dih-tor-ee ______
19. mir-IN-goh-plass-tee ______
20. VER-tih-goh ______
21. tim-pah-NOM-eh-tree ______
22. oh-TYE-tis ______
23. oh-TOL-oh-jist ______
24. tin-EYE-tus ______
25. AW-dee-oh-gram ______

WORKSHEET 13E

Word Search Puzzle

Directions: Find and circle the answer for each fill-in-the-blank question in the word search puzzle.

L	A	M	J	M	C	J	Y	M	M	T	R	X
P	N	S	K	H	X	I	M	H	C	K	W	M
H	I	B	T	N	Y	S	T	A	G	M	U	S
O	E	X	K	I	K	K	R	S	N	V	L	K
T	C	R	V	T	G	A	N	D	U	M	Y	L
O	S	A	D	H	T	M	D	C	S	O	G	R
P	E	E	M	A	J	L	A	U	V	L	C	L
H	R	L	C	Y	C	N	T	T	A	D	P	A
O	O	H	B	W	F	I	Q	U	I	C	P	J
B	U	C	N	Q	N	W	C	N	C	S	D	J
I	L	O	M	N	P	O	T	W	Q	L	M	L
A	F	C	I	C	M	N	E	L	L	E	N	S
H	L	T	L	A	I	P	O	R	E	P	Y	H

1. ______________ is a bright green dye used to highlight corneal abrasions.
2. A(n) ______________ causes the lens to become opaque or cloudy.
3. Jerky involuntary eye movements are called ______________.
4. ______________ actually means an excessive sensitivity to light.
5. An increase in intraocular pressure may cause ______________.
6. A(n) ______________ chart is used to test visual acuity.
7. Farsightedness is also called ______________.
8. A(n) ______________ neuroma is a benign tumor of the auditory nerve sheath.
9. A(n) ______________ implant is a hearing device surgically placed behind the ear.
10. The medical term for ringing in the ears is ______________.

WORKSHEET 13F

Crossword Puzzle

Directions: Use the definitions to complete the crossword puzzles.

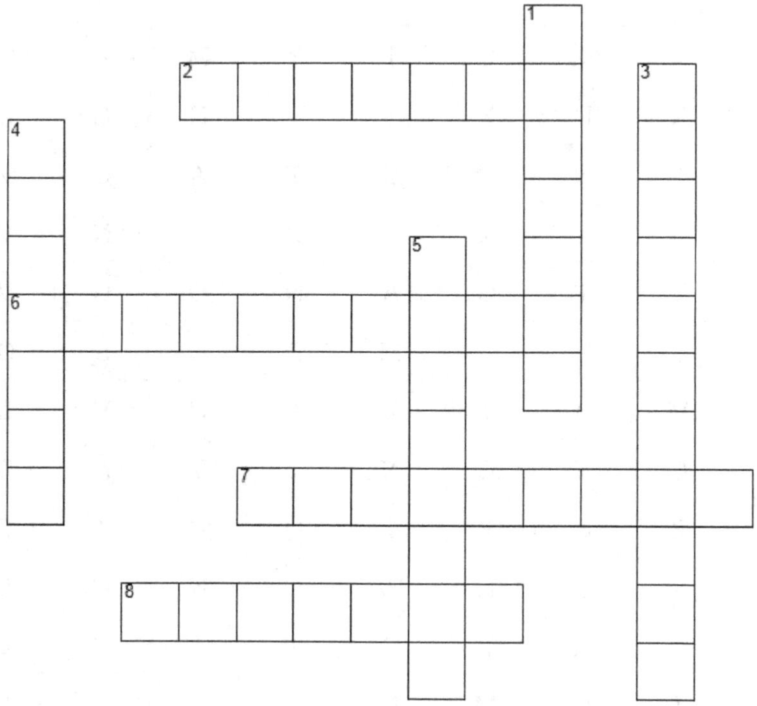

ACROSS

2 Inner ear structure shaped like a snail shell

6 The ______________ tube connects the middle ear to the nasopharynx

7 Term meaning "study of hearing"

8 Common name for tympanic membrane

DOWN

1 ______________ test evaluates balance and equilibrium

3 Term meaning "eardrum record"

4 Otitis ______________ is also called swimmer's ear

5 Ringing in the ears

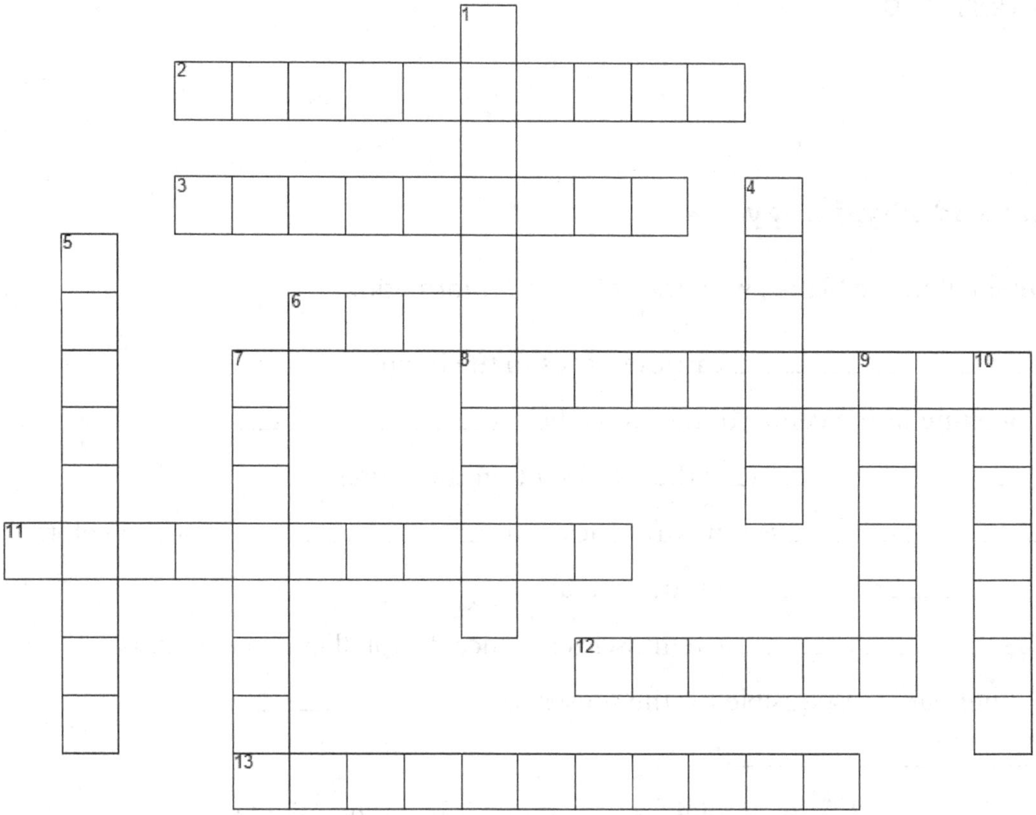

ACROSS

2 Night-blindness

3 Also called lazy eye

6 Also called hordeolum

8 Condition caused by weakness of external eye muscle

11 Mucous membrane protecting anterior eyeball

12 Outer layer of eyeball

13 Condition caused by irregular curvature of cornea

DOWN

1 Bright green dye

4 Visual ____________________ measures sharpness of vision

5 Farsightedness

7 Condition caused by increased intraocular pressure

9 Nearsightedness

10 A(n) ____________________ chart is used to test visual acuity

WORKSHEET 13G

Chapter Review

Anatomy and Physiology

Directions: Fill in the blanks with the requested information.

1. The ____________________ carries images to the brain.
2. The opening in the center of the iris is the ____________________.
3. The ____________________ is the blind spot on the retina.
4. ____________________ see in gray tones and ____________________ see in color.
5. The ____________________ produces tears.
6. The ____________________ eye muscles produce diagonal eye movements.
7. The inner ear is responsible for the senses of ____________________ and ____________________.
8. The ____________________ divides the outer ear from the middle ear.
9. The incus, malleus, and stapes are collectively called the ____________________.
10. The ____________________ is a fluid-filled cavity within the temporal bone.

Word Building

Directions: Build a term for each of the following items.

1. drooping eyelid ____________________
2. paralysis of ciliary body ____________________
3. double vision ____________________
4. pertaining to within eye ____________________
5. softening of sclera ____________________
6. retina disease ____________________
7. incision into eardrum ____________________
8. surgical repair of ear ____________________
9. instrument to measure hearing ____________________
10. eustachian tube inflammation ____________________

Matching

Directions: Match the term with its definition.

_____ **1.** nyctalopia	**a.** Dry eyes
_____ **2.** presbyopia	**b.** Ringing in the ears
_____ **3.** optician	**c.** Eye tumor in children
_____ **4.** papilledema	**d.** Sensitivity to strong light
_____ **5.** xerophthalmia	**e.** Middle ear infection
_____ **6.** achromatopsia	**f.** Increase in intraocular pressure
_____ **7.** photophobia	**g.** Procedure to treat myopi
_____ **8.** amblyopia	**h.** Night blindness
_____ **9.** myopia	**i.** Sharpness of vision
_____ **10.** glaucoma	**j.** Lazy eye
_____ **11.** cataract	**k.** Looks for corneal abrasions
_____ **12.** retinoblastoma	**l.** Grinds corrective lens
_____ **13.** hordeolum	**m.** Dizziness
_____ **14.** blepharoptosis	**n.** A stye
_____ **15.** strabismus	**o.** Loss of vision with aging
_____ **16.** fluorescein staining	**p.** Ear wax
_____ **17.** visual acuity	**q.** Drooping eyelid
_____ **18.** binaural	**r.** Allows drainage of fluid from middle ear
_____ **19.** tinnitus	**s.** Choked disk
_____ **20.** cerumen	**t.** Opaque lens
_____ **21.** vertigo	**u.** Dilates the pupil
_____ **22.** PE tubes	**v.** Nearsightedness
_____ **23.** OM	**w.** Referring to both ears
_____ **24.** LASIK	**x.** Color blindness
_____ **25.** mydriatic	**y.** Caused by eye muscle weakness

QUIZ 13A

New Word Parts Quiz

Directions: Define the combining form or suffix in the spaces provided.

1. blephar/o ____________________
2. chromat/o ____________________
3. core/o ____________________
4. cycl/o ____________________
5. dipl/o ____________________
6. glauc/o ____________________
7. irid/o ____________________
8. kerat/o ____________________
9. lacrim/o ____________________
10. ocul/o ____________________
11. papill/o ____________________
12. phac/o ____________________
13. presby/o ____________________
14. uve/o ____________________
15. vitre/o ____________________
16. audi/o ____________________
17. aur/o ____________________
18. acous/o ____________________
19. myring/o ____________________
20. staped/o ____________________
21. salping/o ____________________
22. tympan/o ____________________
23. -opia ____________________
24. –metrist ____________________
25. -cusis ____________________

QUIZ 13B

Labeling Diagram

Directions: Label the structures of the eye.

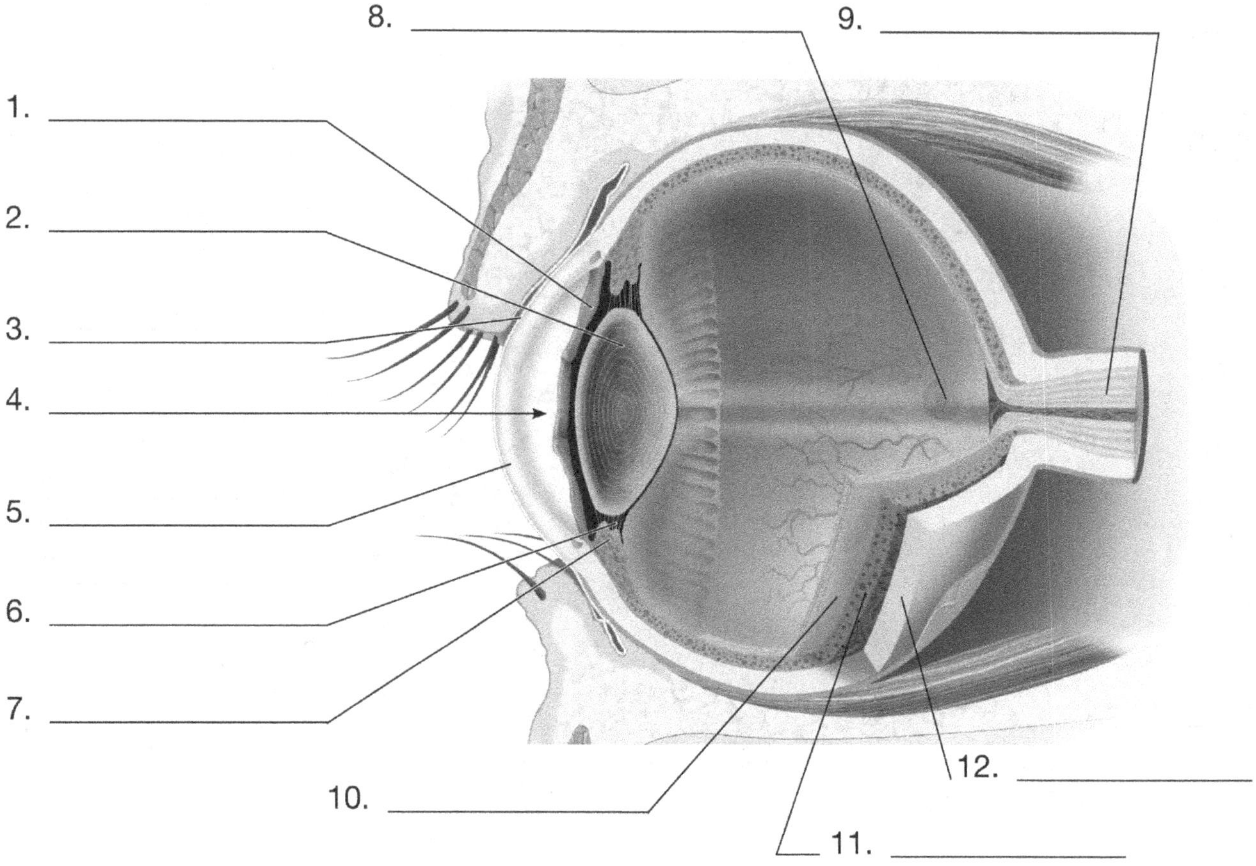

QUIZ 13C

Labeling Diagram

Directions: Label the structures of the ear.

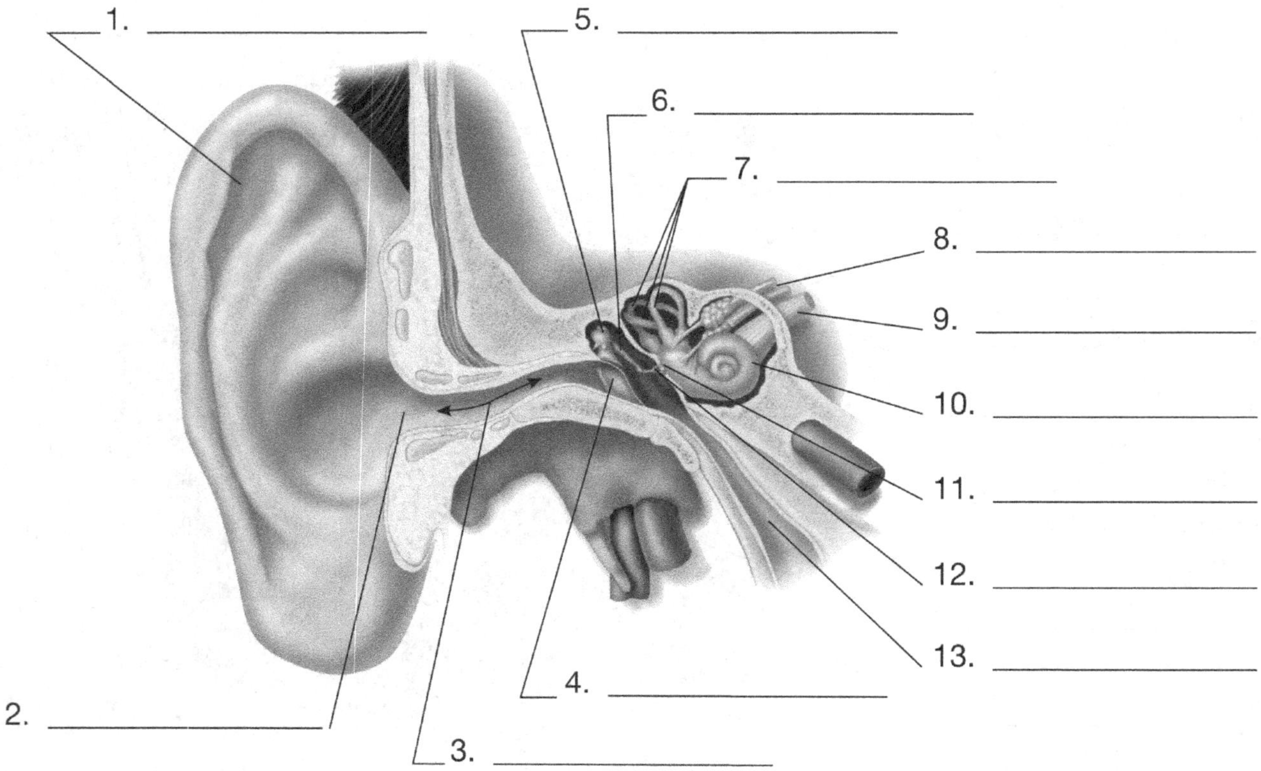

QUIZ 13D

New Word Building Quiz

Directions: Build a single medical term for each phrase below.

1. pertaining to the conjunctiva ____________________
2. pertaining to the cornea ____________________
3. pertaining to the iris ____________________
4. pertaining to tears ____________________
5. pertaining to the eye ____________________
6. pertaining to the pupil ____________________
7. pertaining to the retina ____________________
8. pertaining to the sclera ____________________
9. inflammation of the choroid ____________________
10. retina disease ____________________
11. one who measures vision ____________________
12. eye paralysis ____________________
13. double vision ____________________
14. removal of eyelid ____________________
15. softening of the sclera ____________________
16. pertaining to hearing ____________________
17. hearing specialist ____________________
18. pertaining to the ear ____________________
19. pertaining to the cochlea ____________________
20. pertaining to the eardrum ____________________
21. small ear condition ____________________
22. ear pain ____________________
23. surgical repair of eardrum ____________________
24. incision into the labyrinth ____________________
25. pus flow from ear ____________________

QUIZ 13E

Abbreviations Quiz

Directions: Write the medical term for which each abbreviation stands.

1. Astigm ________________
2. EM ________________
3. EOM ________________
4. IOP ________________
5. LASIK ________________
6. PRK ________________
7. REM ________________
8. ET ________________
9. VA ________________
10. XT ________________
11. VF ________________
12. PERRLA ________________
13. Ophth ________________
14. ASL ________________
15. EENT ________________
16. Oto ________________
17. PE tube ________________
18. OM ________________
19. Hz ________________
20. BC ________________

QUIZ 13F

Chapter Review

PART I: Multiple Choice

Directions: Circle the correct answer.

1. The outermost layer of the eye, referred to as the "white" of the eye, is the

a. sclera. **c.** iris.
b. choroid. **d.** pupil.

2. The medical term for nearsightedness is

a. astigmatism. **c.** myopia.
b. hyperopia. **d.** presbyopia.

3. The condition characterized by an increase in intraocular pressure is

a. cataract. **c.** trachoma.
b. strabismus. **d.** glaucoma.

4. The term for involuntary, jerky movements of the eye is

a. glaucoma. **c.** myopia.
b. nystagmus. **d.** strabismus.

5. The medical term for pinkeye is

a. retinitis. **c.** blepharitis.
b. scleritis. **d.** conjunctivitis.

6. The medical term for normal vision is

a. hyperopia. **c.** emmetropia.
b. myopia. **d.** presbyopia.

7. Which of the following is *not* one of the ossicles of the ear?

a. utricle. **c.** incus.
b. malleus. **d.** stapes.

8. The medical term *anacusis* means
   a. pain in the ear.
   b. impairment of hearing.
   c. absence of hearing.
   d. hearing loss due to aging.
9. In conductive hearing loss,
   a. the sound is conducted normally through the external and middle ear but defective in the inner ear.
   b. sound transmission is blocked in the middle and outer ear.
   c. sound transmission is blocked in the middle and inner ear.
   d. sound is conducted normally through the external ear but defective in the middle and the inner ear.
10. The medical term for ringing in the ears is
   a. vertigo.
   b. tinnitus.
   c. hertz.
   d. hordeolum.

PART II: Matching

Directions: Match the term with its definition.

_____ 1. enucleation
_____ 2. antiemetic
_____ 3. cochlear implant
_____ 4. labyrinthitis
_____ 5. otosclerosis
_____ 6. radial keratotomy
_____ 7. Snellen chart
_____ 8. hemianopia
_____ 9. scleral buckling
_____ 10. pterygium

a. Treatment for sensorineural hearing loss
b. Treatment for myopia
c. Hypertrophied conjunctiva
d. Surgical removal of eyeball
e. Treatment for detached retina
f. Loss of half the visual field
g. Inner ear infection
h. Test for visual acuity
i. Treats nausea
j. Loss of mobility of stapes